MRCP 1
300 BEST OF FIVE
QUESTIONS AND
ANSWERS

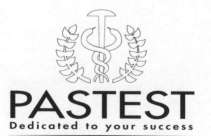

PASTEST
Dedicated to your success

MRCP 1
300 BEST OF FIVE
QUESTIONS AND
ANSWERS

edited by

Wellcome Senior Clinical Fellow
Geraint Rees MRCP PhD
Institute of Cognitive Neuroscience,
University College London,
London WC1N 3AR

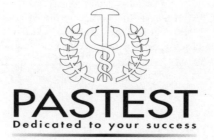

PASTEST
Dedicated to your success

© 2003 PASTEST LTD
Egerton Court
Parkgate Estate
Knutsford
Cheshire
WA16 8DX

Telephone:01565 752000

First published 2003
Reprinted 2004

ISBN:1 901198 979

A catalogue record for this book is available from the British Library.

The information contained within this book was obtained by the authors from
reliable sources. However, while every effort has been made to ensure its
accuracy, no responsibility for loss, damage or injury occasioned to any person
acting or refraining from action as a result of information contained herein can
be accepted by the publishers or authors.

PasTest Revision Books and Intensive Courses
PasTest has been established in the field of postgraduate medical education
since 1972, providing revision books and intensive study courses for doctors
preparing for their professional examinations. Books and courses are
available for the following specialties:

**MRCS, MRCP Part 1 and 2, MRCPCH Part 1 and 2, MRCPsych, MRCOG,
DRCOG, MRCGP, DCH, FRCA, PLAB.**

For further details contact:
**PasTest, Freepost, Knutsford, Cheshire WA16 7BR
Tel:01565 752000   Fax:01565 650264
Email: enquiries@pastest.co.uk   Website:www.pastest.co.uk**

Text prepared by Saxon Graphics Ltd, Derby
Printed and bound by MPG Books Ltd, Bodmin, Cornwall

CONTENTS

CONTRIBUTORS

Cardiology
Dr John Paisey, BM MRCP, Southampton General Hospital, Southampton

Clinical Pharmacology
Dr W Stephen Waring, BMedSci MRCP, Lecturer and Honorary Specialist Registrar, University of Edinburgh, Edinburgh

Dermatology
Dr Mozheh Zamiri, MBChB BSc Hons MRCP, Specialist Registrar in Dermatology, Southern General Hospital, Glasgow

Endocrinology
Dr Anna Crown, MA MBChir MRCP PhD, Specialist Registrar in Endocrinology and Diabetes, Bristol Royal Infirmary, Bristol, URC Neuroendocrinology, Bristol

Gastroenterology
Dr Guruprasad P Aithal, MD MRCP PhD, Consultant Hepatobiliary Physician, Queen's Medical Centre, University Hospital, Nottingham

Haematology
Dr Mary Frances McMullin, MD FRCP (Edin) FRCPath FRCPI, Reader/Consultant Haematologist, Belfast City Hosptial, Belfast

Infectious Diseases
Dr Ian Cropley, Consultant in Infectious Diseases and HIV, Royal Free Hospital, London

Nephrology
Dr Richard Smith, MRCP MD, Consultant Senior Lecturer in Renal Medicine, Bristol

Neurology
Dr Geraint Rees, MRCP PhD, Wellcome Senior Clinical Fellow, Institute of Cognitive Neuroscience, University College London, London

Ophthalmology
Mr David A R Bessant, MD FRCOphth, Locum Consultant Ophthalmologist, Moorfields Eye Hospital, London

Psychiatry
Dr Mo Zoha, MBChB MRCPsych, Consultant Psychiatrist, St Charles Hospital, London

Respiratory Medicine
Dr Howard Branley MBChB MSc MRCP,Clinical Research Fellow, Department of Respiratory Medicine, National Heart & Lung Institute, Imperial College of Science, Technology and Medicine. London

Rheumatology
Dr K Binymin MBChB MRCP MSc, Consultant Physician and Rheumatologist, Southport and Formby General Hospital, Southport

Statistics
Dr A Wade, Senior Lecturer in Medical Statistics, Department of Epidemiology and Public Health, Institute of Child Health, London

INTRODUCTION

The MRCP Part 1 examination consists of two papers, each lasting three hours. Both papers contain 100 'Best of Five' questions (one answer is chosen from five options). Questions in each specialty are randomized across both papers. *No marks are deducted for a wrong answer.*

This book contains 300 questions and expanded answers. It provides up-to-the-minute material in all specialties to give the busy MRCP 1 candidate essential practice before sitting the examination. The questions have excellent clinical scenarios encountered in everyday hospital practice. The expanded answers provide detailed teaching notes to aid revision.

One-best from five answer questions test application and problem-solving unlike true/false MCQs, which tested the recall of knowledge. In order to answer one-best of five questions correctly, it is necessary to apply basic knowledge – not just be able to remember it. A good strategy that can be used with many well-written one-best of five MCQs is to try to reach the correct answer without first scrutinizing the five options.

By working through these questions and answers candidates can also highlight subjects that need further revision. These subjects are covered in detail in *Essential Revision Notes for MRCP* by Philip Kalra. Use both books together to help you pass the MRCP 1 exam.

NORMAL VALUES

Blood, serum and plasma
Haematology

Haemoglobin	12.5–14.5 g/dl
Mean corpuscular volume (MCV)	80–96 fl
Mean corpuscular haemoglobin (MCH)	28–32 pg
Mean corpuscular haemoglobin concentration (MCHC)	32–35 g/dl
White cell count (WCC)	$4–11 \times 10^9/l$
Differential WCC: Neutrophils	$1.5–7 \times 10^9/l$
Lymphocytes	$1.5–4 \times 10^9/l$
Eosinophils	$0.04–0.4 \times 10^9/l$
Platelet count	$150–400 \times 10^9/l$
Reticulocyte count	$50–100 \times 10^9/l$
Prothrombin time (PT)	12–17 s
Activated partial thromboplastin time (APTT)	24–38 s
Thrombin time (TT)	14–22 s
Fibrinogen	2–5 g/l
Fibrinogen degradation products (FDP)	< 10 μg/ml
International normalised ratio (INR)	< 1.4
Iron (Fe^{2+})	14–29 μmol/l
Total iron-binding capacity (TIBC)	45–72 μmol/l
Ferritin	15–200 μg/l
Vitamin B_{12}	120–700 pmol/l
Folate (serum)	2.0–11.0 μg/l
Red cell folate	160–640 μg/l
Erythrocyte sedimentation rate (ESR)	< 12 mm/hour
Plasma viscosity	1.5–1.72 cP

Immunology/Rheumatology

C-reactive protein (CRP)	< 5 mg/l
IgG	6.0–13.0 g/l
IgM	0.4–2.5 g/l
IgA	0.8–3.0 g/l

Endocrinology

Fasting glucose	3.0–6.0 mmol/l
Hb A$_{1c}$	3.8–6.4%
Thyroid stimulating hormone (TSH)	0.3–4.0 mU/l
Thyroxine(T4)	58–174 nmol/l
Free T4 (FT4)	10–24 pmol/l
Parathyroid hormone (PTH)	0.8–8.0 pmol/l

Biochemistry

Sodium (Na$^+$)	137–144 mmol/l
Potassium (K$^+$)	3.5–4.9 mmol/l
Chloride	95–107 mmol/l
Urea	0–180 μmol/l
Creatinine	60–110 μmol/l
Calcium (Ca^{2+}), corrected	2.25–2.70 mmol/l
Phosphate	0.8–1.4 mmol/l
Creatine kinase (CK)	< 120 U/l
Uric acid	0–0.43 mmol/l
Copper	12–26 μmol/l
Caeruloplasmin	200–350 mg/l
Amylase	60–180 U/l
Alanine aminotransferase (ALT)	5–35 U/l
Aspartate aminotransferase (AST)	1–31 U/l
Alkaline phosphatase (ALP)	20–120 U/l
Lactate dehydrogenase (LDH)	10–250 U/l
Gamma-glutamyl transferase (GGT)	4–35 U/l (<50 U/l in men)
Bilirubin (total)	1–22 μmol/l
Total protein	61–76 g/l
Albumin	37–49 g/l
Cholesterol	< 5.2 mmol/l
Triglyceride (fasting)	0.45–1.69 mmol/l

Blood gases

pH	7.36–7.44
PaO$_2$	11.3–12.6 kPa
PaCO$_2$	4.7–6.0 kPa
Bicarbonate	20–28 mmol/l

Therapeutic drug levels

Digoxin (≥6 h post-dose)	1–2 μg/l
Lithium	0.4–1.0 mmol/l

Urine

Albumin/creatinine ratio (random sample)   < 2.5 mg/mmol
Total protein   < 0.2 g/24 h
Glomerular filtration rate (GFR)   70–140 ml/min

Cerebrospinal fluid (CSF)

Opening pressure   5–18 cmH$_2$O
Total protein   0.15–0.45 g/l
Glucose   3.3–4.4 mmol/l
Cell count   < 5 cells/mm^3
Differential cell count: Lymphocytes   60–70%
Monocytes   30–50%
Neutrophils   None

Questions

1. A 46-year-old man is admitted with an episode of chest pain and breathlessness. On admission an ECG shows anterior ST elevation and he receives thrombolysis with rt-PA and makes a good recovery. Admission blood tests: Renal function normal, FBC normal, cholesterol 5.5 mmol/l, triglycerides 3.2 mmol/l. Which one of the following is the most appropriate combination of drugs on discharge?

    ☐ A   Losartan, bezafibrate, aspirin, diltiazem
    ☐ B   Losartan, simvastatin, clopidogrel, atenolol
    ☐ C   Ramipril, bezafibrate, aspirin, atenolol
    ☐ D   Ramipril, simvastatin, aspirin, atenolol
    ☐ E   Ramipril, simvastatin, warfarin, atenolol

2. A 36-year-old woman consults her GP, concerned about hirsutism. On questioning, she says that her periods have always been irregular and the length of her menstrual cycle varies from 21 to 42 days. Her body mass index is 28 kg/m². Other than some dark hairs on her upper lip and chin, the physical examination is unremarkable. Which one of the following is the most likely diagnosis?

    ☐ A   Cushing's syndrome
    ☐ B   Premature menopause
    ☐ C   Primary hypothyroidism
    ☐ D   A virilising tumour
    ☐ E   Polycystic ovarian syndrome

3. A 58-year-old woman is brought to the Accident and Emergency Department unresponsive after collapsing at her home. Her husband reports that she felt well that morning, but developed a progressively severe headache. She has a history of hypertension and atrial fibrillation for which she is anticoagulated. On examination she has a blood pressure of 220/140 mmHg and has apnoea alternating with hyperpnoea. She responds only to noxious stimuli, with right-sided extensor posturing. She has papilloedema and an unreactive pupil on the left, diffuse hyper-reflexia and bilateral upgoing plantars. Which one of the following herniation syndromes is most consistent with her clinical presentation?

☐ **A** Cingulate gyrus beneath the falx
☐ **B** Temporal lobe uncus across the tentorium
☐ **C** Diencephalon through the tentorial notch
☐ **D** Brainstem through the tentorial notch
☐ **E** Cerebellar tonsils through the foramen magnum

4. Bioavailability is an important factor determining the extent to which an orally administered drug will be effective. Which one of the following factors is thought NOT to influence bioavailability of an orally administered drug?

☐ **A** Extent of protein binding
☐ **B** Formulation of the drug
☐ **C** Hepatic impairment
☐ **D** Rate of gastric emptying
☐ **E** Sensitivity of the drug to acid hydrolysis

5. A 24-year-old man presents with a four-day history of a worsening skin eruption preceded by symptoms of headache, fever and arthralgia. On examination, there is evidence of a widespread purpuric rash affecting the extensor aspects of his forearms, legs and buttocks. Investigations demonstrate a raised white cell count with a neutrophilia, and a raised serum IgA level. Urinalysis reveals microscopic haematuria and proteinuria. What is the most likely diagnosis?

☐ A Pigmented purpuric dermatosis
☐ B Linear IgA disease
☐ C Rheumatic fever
☐ D Henoch-Schönlein purpura
☐ E Erythema multiforme

6. A 35-year-old woman attends her regular medical clinic. The physician notes that she is anaemic and further investigation reveals the following results: haemoglobin 6.5 g/dl, MCV 76 fl, MCH 28 pg, MCHC 33 g/dl, WCC 8.5 × 10⁹/l with a normal differential, platelets 505 × 10⁹/l, serum iron 12 μmol/l (normal range 14–29 μmol/l), TIBC 40 μmol/l (normal range 45–72 μmol/l), ferritin 250 μg/l (normal range 15–200 μg/l). What is the most likely cause of her anaemia?

☐ A Sideroblastic anaemia
☐ B Iron deficiency anaemia
☐ C Thalassaemia trait
☐ D Anaemia of chronic disease
☐ E Lead poisoning

7. A 70-year-old man presents with a four-day history of increasing confusion, headache and fever. He is not displaying any signs of meningism. A contrast-enhanced CT scan is unremarkable. Magnetic resonance imaging (MRI) shows a high signal on T2-weighted images in the left frontal lobe. A lumbar puncture shows clear CSF, with 80 white blood cells/mm^3 (95% lymphocytes), protein 0.7 g/l and an opening pressure of 22 cm. No organisms are seen on Gram staining and there was insufficient CSF taken for glucose estimation. What is the most likely causative organism?

☐ A *Borrelia burgdorferi*
☐ B *Treponema pallidum*
☐ C Herpes simplex virus (HSV) type 1
☐ D *Listeria monocytogenes*
☐ E *Mycobacterium tuberculosis*

8. A 26-year-old diabetic woman is found to have bilateral retinal haemorrhages, microaneurysms and intraretinal microvascular anomalies during the first trimester of pregnancy. Which one of the following statements is true?

☐ A She should have an ophthalmic review weekly during her pregnancy
☐ B These features are consistent with preproliferative diabetic retinopathy
☐ C She should be treated with panretinal laser photocoagulation
☐ D She should be treated with focal laser photocoagulation
☐ E Progression of retinopathy is unlikely at this stage

9. A 58-year-old widower describes the distressing experience of hearing the voice of his dead wife berating him. Which one of the following characteristics would most support defining this experience as a pseudohallucination?

☐ A The voice is located in subjective space
☐ B The voice is of a deceased person
☐ C The voice is subject to conscious control
☐ D The voice speaks directly to the patient
☐ E The voice does not speak directly to the patient

10. A 77-year-old patient presents with lethargy, nausea and vomiting and is found to have a creatinine of 652 μmol/l, urea of 44.3 mmol/l, Na$^+$ of 134 mmol/l, K$^+$ of 5.9 mmol/l and a haemoglobin of 11.6 g/dl. On examination, blood pressure is 146/84 mmHg and his bladder is palpable to the umbilicus. Ultrasound scan confirms a large bladder with a 5.9-cm diameter prostate, bilateral pelvicalyceal dilatation and renal cortical thinning. He is catheterised and passes 7 litres of urine in the first 24 hours. Repeat biochemistry results: creatinine 547 μmol/l, urea 42.1 mmol/l, sodium 123 mmol/l and potassium 5.6 mmol/l. Blood pressure is now 123/54 mmHg lying, falling to 110/45 mmHg on standing. What is the most appropriate management of this patient?

- ☐ A Immediate haemodialysis
- ☐ B Restriction of water intake to 2 litres per day
- ☐ C Hydrocortisone replacement
- ☐ D Correction of hyponatraemia with twice-normal saline as soon as possible
- ☐ E Intravenous normal saline to maintain a CVP of 6–10 cmH$_2$O

11. A 74-year-old man with cryptogenic fibrosing alveolitis is brought to the Accident and Emergency Department with severe dyspnoea. He is known to have moderately severe disease and his last lung function tests showed a forced vital capacity of 60% predicted with a gas transfer factor (TLCO) of 45% predicted. Which one of the following blood gas values (on room air) would fit best with this patient's clinical scenario?

- ☐ A pH 7.10, PaCO$_2$ 9.8 kPa, PaO$_2$ 9.1 kPa, bicarbonate 45 mmol/l
- ☐ B pH 7.24, PaCO$_2$ 8.3 kPa, PaO$_2$ 7.1 kPa, bicarbonate 38 mmol/l
- ☐ C pH 7.38, PaCO$_2$ 5.3 kPa, PaO$_2$ 8.1 kPa, bicarbonate 30 mmol/l
- ☐ D pH 7.52, PaCO$_2$ 2.0 kPa, PaO$_2$ 11.1 kPa, bicarbonate 20 mmol/l
- ☐ E pH 7.54, PaCO$_2$ 3.2 kPa, PaO$_2$ 8.1 kPa, bicarbonate 24 mmol/l

12. A 66-year-old woman has a 15-year history of aggressive deforming rheumatoid arthritis (RA). She has chronic neck pain. She is maintained on D-penicillamine. Two weeks ago she noticed increased difficulty in climbing stairs and three days before admission she was unable to comb her hair or feed herself. Neurological assessment reveals grade 3/5 weakness in both upper and lower limb muscle groups; touch and pinprick sensation were intact, tendon reflexes normal. The Babinski sign is positive bilaterally. Which one of the following tests is MOST appropriate at this stage?

- [ ] **A** Plain X-ray of the cervical spine
- [ ] **B** Electromyography (EMG)
- [ ] **C** Nerve conduction study (NCS)
- [ ] **D** Isotope bone scan
- [ ] **E** Magnetic resonance imaging (MRI) of the cervical spine

13. A 51-year-old lady with type 2 diabetes of 12 years' duration was referred to the Liver Clinic with raised liver enzymes. She is obese and weighs 108 kg. She has been on metformin in the past and has been started on insulin recently because of poor glycaemic control. Her current medications include atenolol for hypertension and imipramine for depression. She consumes alcohol on social occasions only. Her investigations reveal: total bilirubin 9 μmol/l, albumin 30 g/l, ALT 387 U/l, ALP 133 U/l, ferritin 443 μg/l, IgG 33.7 g/l, IgA 1.76 g/l, IgM 1.22 g/l, ANA positive at 1/400, SMA positive at 1/400, hepatitis B and C serology negative. Ultrasound abdomen: diffusely hyperechoic liver, otherwise normal. Which one of the following conclusions is true with regards to the clinical scenario?

- [ ] **A** *HFE* genotyping is indicated to confirm the diagnosis
- [ ] **B** Ultrasonographic features are specific for non-alcoholic steatohepatitis (NASH)
- [ ] **C** Antidepressants should be withdrawn and liver enzymes should be monitored
- [ ] **D** Liver biopsy would show features of bridging necrosis
- [ ] **E** Serological pattern is diagnostic of systemic lupus erythematosus

14. A 60-year-old right-handed woman is admitted with loss of power and sensation in the right arm and leg, associated with word-finding difficulty. Physical examination confirms these findings and reveals a right carotid bruit and normal heart sounds. The neurological signs resolve over the two hours after admission. Her GP letter states that she has paroxysmal atrial fibrillation and that she had a duodenal ulcer treated with triple therapy five years ago. She takes no regular medication. Which one of the following treatments is the most appropriate for secondary prevention of transient ischaemic attacks?

- [ ] **A** Aspirin
- [ ] **B** Aspirin, dipyridamole and omeprazole
- [ ] **C** Clopidogrel
- [ ] **D** Aspirin and omeprazole
- [ ] **E** Warfarin to an INR of 2–3.5

15. A 54-year-old woman is treated with oral amoxicillin 500 mg thrice daily for five days. Her respiratory symptoms improve, but she develops profuse diarrhoea associated with fever. On examination the pulse rate is 98 bpm, blood pressure 136/80 mmHg, with generalised abdominal tenderness. Stool culture is strongly positive for *Clostridium difficile* and you suspect a diagnosis of pseudomembranous colitis. Which one of the following treatments would be most appropriate?

- [ ] **A** Ciprofloxacin
- [ ] **B** Co-amoxiclav
- [ ] **C** Erythromycin
- [ ] **D** Metronidazole
- [ ] **E** Trimethoprim

16. One hundred children with fragile X syndrome have their heights measured and these are expressed as sd scores (i.e. they are corrected for age). The mean score is −0.8 and standard deviation 0.15. On the basis of this sample, what is the 95% confidence interval for the population average sd score?

☐ A (−0.5 to 1.1)
☐ B −0.8
☐ C (−0.496 to 1.087)
☐ D (−0.83 to −0.77)
☐ E (−0.845 to −0.765)

17. A 27-year-old woman presents with a two-month history of an asymptomatic red eruption affecting her right hand. It has been slowly increasing in size over this time, and is spreading outwards in a circular pattern. She also suffers from type 1 diabetes mellitus. On examination, there is a 2-cm circle of closely-set, small, smooth firm red papules on the dorsum of the right hand, with no overlying scale. What is the most likely diagnosis?

☐ A Necrobiosis lipoidica
☐ B Diabetic dermopathy
☐ C Granuloma annulare
☐ D Diabetic bullae
☐ E Tinea infection

18. 'Screening bloods' are taken from an 80-year-old lady, admitted after a fall. The results included: corrected calcium 2.85 mmol/l, urea and electrolytes normal.

Subsequently, her parathyroid hormone concentration is found to be 12 pmol/l (normal range 0.8–8 pmol/l). Which one of the following is the most likely diagnosis?

☐ A Hypercalcaemia of malignancy
☐ B Primary hyperparathyroidism
☐ C Osteomalacia
☐ D Secondary hyperparathyroidism
☐ E Myeloma

19. A 75-year-old lady presents with increasing tiredness for six months. On examination she is pale and has 6 cm of splenomegaly. Her haemoglobin is 7.2 gl/dl, MCV 85 fl, WCC 21.5 × 10⁹/l and platelets 45 × 10⁹/l. Examination of her blood film reveals teardrop-shaped red cells and occasional nucleated red cells. Biochemistry is as follows: urea 8.5 mmol/l, creatinine 175 μmol/l, AST 25 U/l, ALT 23 U/l ALP 98 U/l, and LDH 1532 U/l. What is the most likely diagnosis?

☐ **A** Acute myeloid leukaemia
☐ **B** Myelofibrosis
☐ **C** Secondary carcinoma infiltrating the spleen
☐ **D** Chronic myeloid leukaemia
☐ **E** Aplastic anaemia

20. A 52-year-old woman presents with a three-month history of right-sided tingling, numbness and weakness. Her entire right side is completely numb, yet hypersensitive to touch. Five years earlier she underwent mastectomy for breast carcinoma. She has a hemiplegic gait, right hemianaesthesia to all sensory modalities, minimal weakness, and flexor plantars. What is the most likely diagnosis?

☐ **A** Right cerebellar infarction
☐ **B** Left postcentral gyrus metastasis
☐ **C** Left posterior cerebral artery infarction
☐ **D** Left thalamic metastasis
☐ **E** Multiple sclerosis

21. A 22-year-old woman presents with night blindness, deafness and cerebellar ataxia. What is the most likely diagnosis?

☐ **A** Usher syndrome
☐ **B** Lawrence-Moon Bardet-Biedl syndrome
☐ **C** Refsum disease
☐ **D** Kearns-Sayre syndrome
☐ **E** Abetalipoproteinaemia

22. A 24-year-old diabetic man presents with a high fever and an exquisitely tender, hot, swollen, erythematous thigh, with marked crepitus extending from the knee to the inguinal ligament. What is the most likely diagnosis?

☐ **A** Infected thrombophlebitis
☐ **B** Staphylococcal abscess of the thigh at an injection site
☐ **C** Rupture of a femoral artery mycotic aneurysm
☐ **D** Necrotising fasciitis
☐ **E** Severe streptococcal cellulitis

23. A 35-year-old woman complains of a number of troublesome symptoms for which no organic cause can be found. She appears upset and you suspect that some, but not all, of her symptoms may be attributable to an anxiety disorder. With this lady which one of the following is least likely to be secondary to anxiety?

☐ **A** Burning on micturition
☐ **B** Chest pain at rest
☐ **C** Constipation
☐ **D** Diarrhoea
☐ **E** Dysphagia

24. A 49-year-old lady is referred to the Accident and Emergency Department by her GP with cough, fever and breathlessness. The GP mentions she has recently had influenza. She has a temperature of 38.9 °C, inspiratory crackles at the left base, and oxygen saturations of 94% on room air. You decide that she has left lower lobe pneumonia. She is not known to have any drug allergies. What would be your antibiotic regimen of choice?

☐ **A** Flucloxacillin
☐ **B** Amoxicillin and flucloxacillin
☐ **C** Ciprofloxacin
☐ **D** Amoxicillin
☐ **E** Erythromycin and rifampicin

25. A 68-year-old woman has a seven-year history of rheumatoid arthritis. She presented with recurrent attacks of red congested eyes, noticed by her husband. She denies any visual symptoms, dry eyes or dry mouth. What is the MOST likely cause for her eye problem?

- [ ] **A** Scleritis
- [ ] **B** Episcleritis
- [ ] **C** Keratitis
- [ ] **D** Uveitis
- [ ] **E** Choroiditis

26. A 17-year-old South Asian girl presents with a febrile illness. It had begun with a sore throat three weeks previously but at the time of presentation has progressed to cause sharp central chest pain and swollen tender left knee and ankle joints. On examination there is a pericardial rub and pansystolic murmur and a slightly raised ring-shaped erythematous rash is seen on the trunk. Blood tests show haemoglobin 9.5 g/dl (normal range 12.5–14.5 g/dl), WCC 12.5 × 10⁹/l (normal range 4–11 × 10⁹/l), platelets 406 × 10⁹/l (normal range 150–400 × 10⁹/l), ESR 120 mm/h (normal range <12 mm/h), CRP 98 mg/l (normal range <5 mg/l), CK 300 U/l (normal range <120 U/l). Chest X-ray shows an enlarged globular heart. Echocardiography shows a moderate pericardial effusion and thickened mitral valve leaflets with mitral regurgitation and globally depressed left ventricular function. Which one of the following is the correct diagnosis?

- [ ] **A** Coxsackie B viral infection
- [ ] **B** Rheumatic fever
- [ ] **C** Sarcoidosis
- [ ] **D** Still's disease
- [ ] **E** Systemic lupus erythematosus

27. A 64-year-old man is admitted for routine hip replacement and is found to have a plasma sodium of 125 mmol/l. He has a history of hypertension, a grand mal convulsion following cerebral infarction, and angina. His medications are carbamazepine, isosorbide mononitrate, atenolol, and simvastatin. What is the most likely cause of his hyponatraemia?

☐ A Pseudohyponatraemia
☐ B Drug-induced nephrogenic diabetes insipidus
☐ C Addison's disease
☐ D Syndrome of inappropriate ADH secretion (SIADH)
☐ E Drug-induced renal sodium loss

28. A 56-year-old lady has recently been diagnosed with angina, and she has been commenced on sublingual glyceryl trinitrate (GTN) spray for symptomatic relief. Which one of the following factors best explains why the sublingual route is preferred?

☐ A Ease of administration
☐ B High first-pass metabolism of orally administered GTN
☐ C High incidence of gastrointestinal symptoms associated with oral preparations
☐ D Less risk of nitrate tolerance than by oral administration
☐ E Orally administered GTN has an onset of action of 4–6 hours

29. A 56-year-old man complains of increased skin fragility and blistering lesions affecting his scalp and the backs of his hands. He admits to drinking 60 units of alcohol per week. On examination, there is evidence of multiple erosions and blisters affecting sun-exposed sites. Milia are present at areas of healed blisters. Investigations reveal: WCC 6.4 × 10⁹/l, haemoglobin 18.5 g/dl, platelets 160 × 10⁹/l, Na⁺ 141 mmol/l, K⁺ 3.9 mmol/l, urea 4.4 mmol/l, creatinine 78 μmol/l, bilirubin 23 μmol/l, AST 55 U/l, ALT 42 U/l, ALP 380 U/l, GGT 80 U/l, ferritin 985 μg/l. Which enzyme is most likely to be reduced in activity in this condition?

☐ A Uroporphyrinogen synthase
☐ B Uroporphyrinogen decarboxylase
☐ C Porphobilinogen deaminase
☐ D Protoporphyrinogen oxidase
☐ E Coproporphyrinogen oxidase

30. A 54-year-old Caucasian man presents with symptoms of heartburn and acid reflux of 2 years' duration. He had a barium swallow one year ago, which demonstrated a hiatus hernia. Subsequently he was treated with ranitidine 300 mg a day, which reduced the heartburn. However, he continued to have breakthrough symptoms. Which one of the following statements is true regarding this patient?

☐ A Reflux of contrast into the oesophagus on barium swallow is diagnostic of gastro-oesophageal reflux disease (GORD)

☐ B Failure of H_2-receptor antagonists to completely resolve symptoms suggests an underlying Barrett's metaplasia

☐ C Endoscopic abnormalities are essential for the diagnosis of gastro-oesophageal reflux disease

☐ D Oesophageal manometry demonstrating low oesophageal sphincter tone is the key to the diagnosis of gastro-oesophageal reflux disease

☐ E 24-hour oesophageal pH study is indicated for the diagnosis of gastro-oesophageal reflux disease in those who have no endoscopic abnormalities

31. A 35-year-old teacher consults her GP. She gave birth to her second child five months ago. When he was three months old, she returned to work and stopped breastfeeding. Since then, she has been feeling anxious and irritable. On examination, the only abnormal finding was a sinus tachycardia. Her GP checked her thyroid function tests, found that she was thyrotoxic and referred her to the Endocrine Clinic. Which one of the following investigations would best distinguish between Graves' disease and postpartum thyroiditis?

☐ A Ultrasound scan of the thyroid
☐ B Thyroid autoantibody titre
☐ C Isotope scan of the thyroid
☐ D CT scan of the neck
☐ E Fine-needle aspiration biopsy of the thyroid

32. A 25-year-old nulliparous woman is involved in a serious road traffic accident. She is undergoing surgery for a ruptured spleen and liver lacerations. Her blood group is A Rh-negative. She was transfused with all the available supplies of O Rh-negative blood while being stabilised in Accident and Emergency and has already been transfused with 10 units of A Rh-negative blood. There is no more A Rh-negative blood available. She continues to bleed profusely and is hypotensive. Which is the best blood group to give her now?

- ☐ **A** AB Rh-positive
- ☐ **B** O Rh-positive
- ☐ **C** B Rh-negative
- ☐ **D** AB Rh-negative
- ☐ **E** A Rh-positive

33. A 34-year-old woman presents complaining of episodic leg weakness and crampy abdominal pain, without diarrhoea. During an episode, her abdomen is distended, with decreased bowel sounds, and she has distal leg weakness with loss of knee and ankle jerks. Which biosynthetic pathway is most likely to be defective?

- ☐ **A** Haem
- ☐ **B** Thyroxine
- ☐ **C** Corticosteroids
- ☐ **D** Glucose
- ☐ **E** Collagen

34. A 77-year-old man complains of recent onset of reduced vision in his left eye, which has a visual acuity of 6/60. Fundoscopy reveals unilateral optic atrophy. What is the most likely cause?

- ☐ **A** Demyelination
- ☐ **B** Leber's optic atrophy
- ☐ **C** Pituitary adenoma
- ☐ **D** Raised intracranial pressure
- ☐ **E** Anterior ischaemic optic neuropathy

35. A 65-year-old Indian woman who has lived in rural northern India until the age of 50, and who has just returned to the UK after a four-week stay back in her home village, develops acute jaundice with an ALT of 3564 U/l following a 'flu-like' illness during the monsoon season. What is the most likely diagnosis?

- ☐ **A** Leptospirosis
- ☐ **B** Yellow fever
- ☐ **C** Acute hepatitis A
- ☐ **D** Acute hepatitis B
- ☐ **E** Acute hepatitis E

36. A 26-year-old inpatient describes being very worried that every time nurses pass by with an injection, that he will rush up, grab the needle and then stab someone. He fails in his attempts not to focus on this and is becoming increasingly distressed. Which one of the following is a recognised description of his complaint?

- ☐ **A** Obsessional doubt
- ☐ **B** Obsessional impulse
- ☐ **C** Obsessional ritual
- ☐ **D** Obsessional rumination
- ☐ **E** Obsessional thought

37. A 47-year-old woman presents complaining of dry eyes and mouth. On direct questioning, a history of Raynaud's phenomenon is elicited. Routine biochemistry demonstrates a sodium of 135 mmol/l, potassium 2.8 mmol/l, creatinine 106 μmol/l, bicarbonate 18 mmol/l, chloride 110 mmol/l. Dipstick urinalysis demonstrates: pH 7, no blood or protein. A urinary acidification test is performed during which the urine pH never falls below 5.4. Which one of the following statements is true?

- ☐ **A** The biochemical abnormalities are due to an inability of the kidney to reabsorb bicarbonate
- ☐ **B** Nephrocalcinosis may occur
- ☐ **C** Osteomalacia may occur
- ☐ **D** There may be an associated Fanconi syndrome
- ☐ **E** May be caused by out-of-date tetracycline

38. A new test is devised that is cheaper than the current alternative for detecting tuberculosis. Out of a sample of 520 patients, 200 are found to be positive for tuberculosis. When the new test is applied, 180 of the confirmed tuberculosis patients test positive as well as 25 of those found not to have the disease using the original test. Which one of the following is the positive predictive value for the new test?

   ☐ A 180/205
   ☐ B 295/320
   ☐ C 475/520
   ☐ D 180/200
   ☐ E 295/315

39. A 39-year-old man with sarcoidosis is admitted to the Accident and Emergency Department with worsening breathlessness. A chest X-ray is reported by the radiologist as stage 3 pulmonary sarcoidosis. Which one of the following patterns is his chest X-ray likely to show?

   ☐ A Bilateral hilar lymphadenopathy
   ☐ B Pleural effusion
   ☐ C Diffuse pulmonary fibrosis
   ☐ D Interstitial infiltrates
   ☐ E Bilateral hilar lymphadenopathy and interstitial infiltrates

40. A 30-year-old woman with a history of recurrent DVT and pulmonary embolism is found to have a prolonged activated partial thromboplastin time (APTT). What is the MOST likely associated abnormality?

   ☐ A Antithrombin III deficiency
   ☐ B Anticardiolipin antibodies
   ☐ C Anti-Scl-70 antibodies
   ☐ D Anti-Ro antibodies
   ☐ E Protein S deficiency

41. A 44-year-old man presents with general malaise, weight loss and itching. Five years ago he was diagnosed as having ulcerative colitis. He has no bowel symptoms and is maintained on mesalazine. In the past, he had been diagnosed with folliculitis for which he had received treatment with minocycline. He drinks about 20 units of alcohol per week and there is no family history of liver or bowel disease. Physical examination revealed no abnormalities. Investigations: total bilirubin 12 μmol/l, albumin 33 g/l, ALT 200 U/l, ALP 1071 U/l, immunoglobulins normal, ANA negative, AMA negative, SMA positive at 1/40. Ultrasound: increased echotexture of the liver; no dilatation of the extra- or intrahepatic bile ducts. Which one of the following is true with regards to this clinical scenario?

- [ ] A Endoscopic retrograde cholangiopancreatography (ERCP) would be diagnostic for primary sclerosing cholangitis (PSC)
- [ ] B cANCA would be positive in more than 75% of patients with PSC
- [ ] C Positive SMA suggests minocycline-induced chronic hepatitis
- [ ] D Cholangiocarcinoma typically complicates longstanding PSC
- [ ] E Patients with PSC have left-sided colitis with minimal risk of colorectal cancer

42. A 65-year-old man with a history of an anterior myocardial infarct ten years previously presents with syncope. He is otherwise asymptomatic and denies having any palpitations. Bloods tests, including cardiac enzymes, are normal; ECG shows loss of R waves in the septal leads. Cardiac catheterisation is performed and shows a blocked left anterior descending artery and an akinetic anterior wall (ejection fraction 0.28). Following investigation what is the most appropriate treatment of his syncope likely to be?

- [ ] A Amiodarone
- [ ] B Carotid endarterectomy
- [ ] C Dual chamber (DDD) pacemaker
- [ ] D Implantable defibrillator
- [ ] E Single chamber (VVI) pacemaker

43. A 66-year-old woman has received multiple short courses of high-dose corticosteroids for exacerbations of chronic obstructive pulmonary disease. Which one of the following is NOT thought to be a recognised pharmacological effect of hydrocortisone?

- [ ] **A** Binding to the mineralocorticoid receptor
- [ ] **B** Hypokalaemic metabolic alkalosis
- [ ] **C** Increased aldosterone production
- [ ] **D** Inhibition of leukocyte adhesiveness
- [ ] **E** Suppression of ACTH secretion

44. A 26-year-old woman is brought to the Accident and Emergency Department having collapsed in a nightclub with a tonic-clonic seizure. On arrival, she is awake and complaining of nausea and headache. She has moderate pyramidal weakness of the right leg. Computed tomography shows bilateral haemorrhagic infarction of the white matter in the left parietal lobe. Which of the following blood vessels is most likely to be occluded?

- [ ] **A** Right anterior cerebral artery
- [ ] **B** Left middle cerebral artery
- [ ] **C** Sagittal sinus
- [ ] **D** Cavernous sinus
- [ ] **E** Left posterior cerebral artery

45. A 45-year-old sales assistant complains of hair loss. She has noticed bald patches developing in different areas of her scalp. She had been diagnosed with pernicious anaemia six years previously. On examination, there are multiple discrete patches of hair loss with no erythema or scaling. There are a few exclamation-mark hairs present at the edges of the areas. What is the most likely diagnosis?

- [ ] **A** Androgenetic alopecia
- [ ] **B** Telogen effluvium
- [ ] **C** Traumatic alopecia
- [ ] **D** Folliculitis decalvans
- [ ] **E** Alopecia areata

46. A 50-year-old man with a long history of poorly controlled hypertension is found to be persistently hypokalaemic, with otherwise normal urea and electrolytes. His only regular medication is amlodipine. Physical examination reveals hypertensive retinopathy, but is otherwise unremarkable. His body mass index is 21 kg/m². Which one of the following investigations would be the best next step in looking for a potentially treatable cause of his hypertension?

☐ **A** Aldosterone:renin ratio
☐ **B** CT scan of the abdomen
☐ **C** 24-hour ambulatory blood pressure monitoring
☐ **D** Echocardiogram
☐ **E** 24-hour urine collection for urinary free cortisol

47. A 60-year-old woman is admitted for elective hip replacement. She is otherwise fit and healthy and has never been in hospital since the delivery of her second child 35 years previously. The operation is uneventful and during the procedure she is transfused with 4 units of fully crossmatched blood. One week later, when being prepared for discharge, she is noted to be jaundiced. Her haemoglobin is then found to be 8.5 g/dl, MCV 101 fl, WCC 10.5 × 10⁹/l and platelets 445 × 10⁹/l. The most likely cause of her jaundice is:

☐ **A** Gallstones
☐ **B** Halothane toxicity
☐ **C** Myelodysplasia
☐ **D** Hepatitis C
☐ **E** Delayed haemolytic transfusion reaction

48. During a routine examination, a 17-year-old is found by his optician to have an elevated white lesion of the retina nasal to the left optic disc. His ophthalmologist diagnoses a retinal astrocytic hamartoma. With what condition are these lesions most commonly associated?

☐ **A** Sturge-Weber syndrome
☐ **B** Neurofibromatosis
☐ **C** Tuberose sclerosis
☐ **D** von Hippel-Lindau syndrome
☐ **E** Juvenile xanthogranuloma

49. A 41-year-old male patient with moderately well controlled epilepsy describes the recent onset of hearing voices and persecutory delusions. You believe he would benefit from medication for this complaint. Which one of the following would be the most appropriate antipsychotic?

☐ **A** Chlorpromazine
☐ **B** Clozapine
☐ **C** Doxepin
☐ **D** Haloperidol
☐ **E** Zotepine

50. A 30-year-old sheep farmer is admitted with a one-week history of dry cough and increasing shortness of breath and a prominent wheeze. The PaO_2 is 8.0 kPa on room air; the heart rate is 120 bpm and the JVP is elevated by 4 cm. Heart sounds are normal. A widespread expiratory wheeze is audible throughout his chest. Chest X-ray shows diffuse bilateral pulmonary infiltrates. He does have risk factors for HIV, but had a negative HIV test two weeks ago. Which is the most likely causative agent?

☐ **A** Severe acute respiratory syndrome (SARS) coronavirus
☐ **B** *Mycoplasma* pneumonia
☐ **C** *Pneumocystis jiroveci (carinii)*
☐ **D** *Coxiella burnetii*
☐ **E** Coxsackievirus

51. An 18-year-old man with asthma is brought to the Accident and Emergency Department with severe shortness of breath. His peak flow is 90 l/min (normally 550–600 l/min), respiratory rate 32/min and auscultation of his chest reveals barely audible breath sounds throughout. His girlfriend says that he has been ventilated before. At which level of arterial blood gas abnormality would you be most likely to call an anaesthetist for an opinion on intubation and ventilation?

☐ **A** pH 7.28, $PaCO_2$ 6.3 kPa, PaO_2 9.1 kPa, bicarbonate 45 mmol/l
☐ **B** pH 7.24, $PaCO_2$ 8.3 kPa, PaO_2 7.1 kPa, bicarbonate 38 mmol/l
☐ **C** pH 7.38, $PaCO_2$ 5.3 kPa, PaO_2 8.1 kPa, bicarbonate 30 mmol/l
☐ **D** pH 7.52, $PaCO_2$ 2.0 kPa, PaO_2 9.1 kPa, bicarbonate 14 mmol/l
☐ **E** pH 7.56, $PaCO_2$ 3.1 kPa, PaO_2 9.6 kPa, bicarbonate 28 mmol/l

52. A 26-year-old woman is found unconscious with no history available. Pulse is 78 bpm, blood pressure 126/78 mmHg and respiration rate 14/minute. The patient is apyrexial. Examination is otherwise unremarkable. Routine investigations demonstrate: haemoglobin 12.4 g/dl, WCC 6.3 × 10⁹/l, platelets 214 × 10⁹/l, sodium 134 mmol/l, potassium 4.2 mmol/l, chloride 101 mmol/l, urea 5.6 mmol/l, creatinine 134 μmol/l and a blood glucose of 4.6 mmol/l. The pH is 7.28 with a bicarbonate of 17 mmol/l. What is the most likely diagnosis?

- [ ] **A** Acute renal failure
- [ ] **B** Paracetamol overdose
- [ ] **C** Tricyclic antidepressant overdose
- [ ] **D** Salicylate overdose
- [ ] **E** Diabetic ketoacidosis

53. A 28-year-old woman developed joint swelling in the hands, excessive fatigue and extreme tiredness over many years. She also has a photosensitive rash on her face. The possibility of systemic lupus erythematosus (SLE) was raised by her doctor. Which one of the following tests when NEGATIVE will virtually exclude the diagnosis of SLE?

- [ ] **A** Antinuclear antibody (ANA)
- [ ] **B** Anti-double-stranded DNA (Anti-dsDNA)
- [ ] **C** Anti-Sm antibodies
- [ ] **D** Anti-histone antibodies
- [ ] **E** Anti-Ro (SSA) antibodies

54. A patient undergoing angioplasty and stenting for a circumflex lesion is commenced on abciximab post-procedure due to the high risk of early thrombosis of his lesion as judged by the operator. Six hours later he develops epistaxis and bleeding from puncture sites. His platelet count is found to be 4 × 10⁹/l. What is the most likely cause of his thrombocytopenia?

- [ ] **A** Decreased production due to marrow toxicity
- [ ] **B** Disseminated intravascular coagulation (DIC)
- [ ] **C** Haemorrhage
- [ ] **D** Immune-mediated thrombocytopenia
- [ ] **E** Myelofibrosis

55. **Which one of the following factors does not influence volume of distribution (V_d) of an orally administered drug?**

☐ **A** Lipid:aqueous solubility coefficient of the drug
☐ **B** Plasma protein binding
☐ **C** Ratio of body fat to muscle
☐ **D** Serum albumin concentration
☐ **E** Dose of drug

56. **A 14-year-old girl has been referred to the Gastroenterology Clinic for advice and counselling. Her father died of colorectal cancer six months ago at the age of 39 years. Which one of the following is true regarding genetic susceptibility to colorectal cancer?**

☐ **A** Familial adenomatous polyposis (FAP) is inherited as an autosomal recessive disorder
☐ **B** Genetic testing for FAP can be performed using DNA from white blood cells obtained by venepuncture
☐ **C** Congenital hypertrophy of the retinal pigment epithelium (CHRPE) is a characteristic feature of Peutz-Jeghers syndrome
☐ **D** Juvenile polyposis results from mutations of DNA mismatch repair genes
☐ **E** Hereditary non-polyposis colorectal cancer (HNPCC) is characterised by cancers in the left side of the colon

57. **A seven-year-old girl attends with several skin problems. She suffers from epilepsy and mental retardation. She has evidence of small oval white patches on her trunk and some nail changes. Her mother has acne-like papules on both cheeks. What are the nail changes most likely to represent?**

☐ **A** Nail pitting
☐ **B** Onycholysis
☐ **C** Subungual fibromas
☐ **D** Beau's lines
☐ **E** Subungual haematomas

58. A 34-year-old vegan presents with a six-week history of distressing paraesthesiae in her hands and legs. Over the last two weeks, her gait has become unsteady and she feels that her legs have become weak. On examination, vibration and joint-position sense is impaired in the lower limbs. Her legs show increased tone, a mild symmetrical proximal loss of power, hyper-reflexia and bilateral extensor plantars. Her gait is ataxic. What nutritional deficiency is the most likely cause of her problems?

- ☐ A Vitamin B_{12} deficiency
- ☐ B Folic acid deficiency
- ☐ C Thiamine deficiency
- ☐ D Pyridoxine deficiency
- ☐ E Iron deficiency

59. A fit and well 20-year-old man with a steady body mass index of 22 kg/m² registers with a new GP and attends for a 'new patient health check'. Dipstick urinalysis reveals glycosuria +++, but is negative for ketones. A random BM stick reading estimates his blood glucose to be 19 mmol/l. He is not unduly surprised, as exactly the same thing happened to his older brother at a similar age, and he (like many of their relatives) is now settled on a diabetic diet. Which one of the following types of diabetes is this likely to be?

- ☐ A Type 1 diabetes
- ☐ B DIDMOAD syndrome
- ☐ C Type 2 diabetes
- ☐ D Maturity-onset diabetes of the young (MODY)
- ☐ E Metabolic syndrome X

60. A three-year-old Asian child is noted to be very pale. The child is otherwise active and well. His haemoglobin is 3.4 g/dl, RBC 2.4 × 10¹²/l, MCV 63 fl, MCH 22 pg, MCHC 28 g/dl, WCC 4.5 × 10⁹/l with a normal differential, platelets 455 × 10⁹/l. What is the most likely diagnosis?

- ☐ A Iron deficiency anaemia
- ☐ B Folic acid deficiency
- ☐ C Acute lymphoblastic leukaemia
- ☐ D Thalassaemia intermedia
- ☐ E Aplastic anaemia

61. A well, 30-year-old homosexual man who has multiple sexual partners attends the Genitourinary Medicine Clinic for a health check. Which investigation is LEAST useful?

☐ **A** HIV antibody testing
☐ **B** Serological testing for syphilis
☐ **C** Testing for past hepatitis A with a view to vaccination
☐ **D** Testing for current and past hepatitis B with a view to vaccination
☐ **E** Serological testing for herpes simplex virus (HSV) IgG

62. A 45-year-old woman presents with a marked right-sided ptosis and failure of upgaze (elevation). What is the most likely diagnosis?

☐ **A** Horner's syndrome
☐ **B** Third cranial nerve palsy
☐ **C** Dystrophia myotonica
☐ **D** Myasthenia gravis
☐ **E** Dysthyroid eye disease

63. A 24-year-old man has been admitted to a medical ward following an asthma attack. After recovery he confides that he has been upset by a number of recent unusual experiences. Which one of the following experiences would lead you most to suspect the presence of schizophrenia?

☐ **A** Visual hallucinations
☐ **B** Delusion of being a gangster
☐ **C** Command hallucinations
☐ **D** Thought echo
☐ **E** Gustatory hallucinations

64. **A 36-year-old computer programmer with sarcoidosis sees you in the Chest Clinic. She has been reading about sarcoidosis on the Internet and wishes to ask you about her long-term prognosis. Which one of the following features would be most likely to give her a worse prognosis?**

☐ **A** Erythema nodosum
☐ **B** Non-caseating granulomata on transbronchial biopsy
☐ **C** Splenomegaly
☐ **D** Bilateral hilar lymphadenopathy
☐ **E** Decreased gas transfer factor

65. **An 18-year-old man presents with severe right loin pain radiating to his groin. Blood pressure is normal. Dipstick urinalysis demonstrates haematuria ++ with no protein detectable. MSU demonstrates 100 RBCs per high-power field but no white cells. Routine investigations are normal. An abdominal X-ray shows three calculi in the right kidney which have a ground-glass appearance. Which one of the following is true?**

☐ **A** Further stone formation may be prevented by D-penicillamine treatment
☐ **B** Acidification of the urine should be undertaken
☐ **C** Bendroflumethiazide (bendrofluazide) may prevent further stone formation
☐ **D** Urinalysis will demonstrate increased urinary excretion of neutral amino acids
☐ **E** Increased fluid intake has no role in the management

66. **A 30-year-old house cleaner presents with a six-month history of swelling and pain involving the distal interphalangeal joints of the hands. Her hands are stiff in early morning but this eases off towards the afternoon. The ESR is 65 mm in the first hour. What is the MOST likely diagnosis?**

☐ **A** Generalised osteoarthritis
☐ **B** Rheumatoid arthritis
☐ **C** Psoriatic arthritis
☐ **D** Systemic lupus erythematosus (SLE)
☐ **E** Gout

67. An 18-year-old woman attends Casualty with fast, regular palpitations. An ECG is recorded and shows a regular rhythm with a rate of 210 bpm and QRS duration of 80 ms. Shortly after admission the tachycardia spontaneously resolves. A resting ECG in sinus rhythm is taken which shows a PR interval of 50 ms and QRS duration of 120 ms with a positive delta wave in V_1.
What is the mechanism of this woman's tachycardia?

- ☐ **A** Atrial fibrillation
- ☐ **B** Atrioventricular nodal re-entry tachycardia
- ☐ **C** Atrioventricular re-entry tachycardia
- ☐ **D** Macro re-entry atrial tachycardia
- ☐ **E** Ventricular re-entry tachycardia

68. A 47-year-old man has suffered from bipolar affective disorder for ten years and takes lithium carbonate 400 mg daily. He presents to the Accident and Emergency Department stating that he has taken 2 g of lithium carbonate four hours earlier. Which one of the following is NOT a recognised feature of acute lithium intoxication?

- ☐ **A** Blurred vision
- ☐ **B** Drowsiness
- ☐ **C** Hypothyroidism
- ☐ **D** Tremor
- ☐ **E** Weight gain

69. A 40-year-old woman is found to have abnormal liver tests at the time of an insurance medical examination. She is asymptomatic and has never consumed excess alcohol. She has no risk factors for viral hepatitis or any family history of liver disease. There are no stigmata of chronic liver disease and abdominal examination is normal. Investigations reveal: total bilirubin 17 μmol/l, albumin 40 g/l, ALT 81 U/l, ALP 376 U/l, IgG 15.7 g/l, IgA 3.6 g/l, IgM 5.1 g/l, ANA negative, antimitochondrial antibodies (AMA) positive at 1/640. Which one of the following is true with regards to the management of this patient?

- [ ] **A** Perivenular granuloma is diagnostic of primary biliary cirrhosis (PBC)
- [ ] **B** Increasing alkaline phosphatase suggests a poor prognosis
- [ ] **C** If symptomatic, steroid therapy is indicated
- [ ] **D** Ursodeoxycholic acid therapy could delay the need for liver transplantation
- [ ] **E** This condition does not recur following liver transplantation

70. A 21-year-old law student presents with moderately severe acne vulgaris, affecting her face, chest and upper back. She has been treated with topical erythromycin and prolonged courses of oral minocycline, lymecycline and erythromycin. She has no other medical history of note. Treatment with isotretinoin (Roaccutane®) is considered. What is the most important issue to discuss?

- [ ] **A** The risk of renal failure
- [ ] **B** The risk of gout
- [ ] **C** Contraception
- [ ] **D** The risk of skeletal hyperostosis
- [ ] **E** The risk of dry skin

71. A 40-year-old man with no past medical history is admitted to the Accident and Emergency Department with cuts and bruises, following a minor road traffic accident. His history is a bit vague, but he apparently drove into the back of a parked car. No significant symptoms or signs are noted by the Casualty Officer, and she is surprised to see that his BM (capillary blood glucose) on admission was 2.0 mmol/l. What is the best next step in the patient's management?

☐ **A** Oral glucose (e.g. Lucozade® drink or dextrose tablets)
☐ **B** A glucagon injection
☐ **C** Infusion of 50% dextrose
☐ **D** Infusion of 10% dextrose
☐ **E** Venous blood sample

72. A 35-year-old migraineur presents with a ten-hour history of headache and right-sided visual disturbance. On examination he has a right inferior homonymous quandrantanopia. Damage to which structure is most likely to have caused his visual problems?

☐ **A** Optic chiasm
☐ **B** Left lateral geniculate nucleus
☐ **C** Left parietal lobe
☐ **D** Left temporal lobe
☐ **E** Left occipital lobe

73. A 45-year-old woman presents with weight loss, sweating and tachycardia. After investigation she is started on propranolol, diazepam and carbimazole. Two months later she presents to Accident and Emergency in a collapsed state. On examination she is pyrexial, and hypotensive and tachycardic. There was nothing else of note on examination. On investigation her results are: haemoglobin 10.5 g/dl, WCC 0.5 × 10^9/l with neutrophils of 0.2 × 10^9/l, platelets 154 × 10^9/l, reticulocytes 64 × 10^9/l (normal range 50–100 × 10^9/l), prothrombin time 16 s (normal range 12–17 s), APTT 31 s (normal range 24–38 s), thrombin time 17 s (normal range 14–22 s), fibrinogen 2.5 g/l (normal range 2–5 g/l). Which one of the following is the most likely cause of her neutropenia?

- [ ] **A** Propranolol
- [ ] **B** Autoimmune neutropenia
- [ ] **C** Diazepam
- [ ] **D** Carbimazole
- [ ] **E** Septicaemia

74. A 55-year-old man with abnormal liver function tests claims that he likes the occasional drink but vehemently denies having an alcohol problem. You elicit an alcohol history. Which one of the following is a recognised feature of the alcohol dependence syndrome?

- [ ] **A** Consumption of > 42 units per week
- [ ] **B** Denial of having an alcohol problem
- [ ] **C** Excessive alcohol consumption from teenage years onwards
- [ ] **D** Experiencing cravings to have a drink
- [ ] **E** Heavy binge drinking at weekends

75. The Microbiology Laboratory reports that an isolate of *Salmonella typhi* is resistant to ciprofloxacin. What is the most likely explanation?

- [ ] **A** DNA-gyrase mutation
- [ ] **B** β-Lactamase activity
- [ ] **C** Decreased bacterial cell wall permeability
- [ ] **D** Membrane transporter system causing drug efflux
- [ ] **E** Alteration of the ribosomal binding site

76. A 60-year-old woman attends the Chest Clinic with progressive, increasing breathlessness. A chest X-ray reveals a pleural effusion that you aspirate in the clinic under local anaesthetic. She returns to the clinic the following week for the results, which show an eosinophilia, decreased pH and decreased glucose. Which one of the following is the most likely diagnosis?

- [ ] **A** Churg-Strauss syndrome
- [ ] **B** Blood in the pleural space
- [ ] **C** Drug-induced pleuritis
- [ ] **D** Asbestos-related pleural effusion
- [ ] **E** Sarcoidosis

77. A 70-year-old woman, known to have polymyalgia rheumatica for two years, is taking non-steroidal anti-inflammatory drugs and steroid tablets. She is found to have a haemoglobin of 10.2 g/dl with a microcytic hypochromic peripheral blood picture. The ESR was raised at 82 mm/h and immunoglobulin levels were raised. Which one of the following factors is NOT likely to be contributory to her raised ESR level?

- [ ] **A** Anaemia
- [ ] **B** Active polymyalgia rheumatica
- [ ] **C** Old age
- [ ] **D** Microcytosis
- [ ] **E** Hypergammaglobulinaemia

78. A 34-year-old man has haematuria detected at a routine insurance medical. He has a blood pressure of 154/88 mmHg and has no family history of renal disease. Plasma creatinine is normal but ultrasound scan demonstrates multiple bilateral renal cysts. Which one of the following statements is correct?

- [ ] **A** His children have a 25% chance of inheriting this disorder
- [ ] **B** Disease is limited to the kidney
- [ ] **C** Mitral stenosis is a recognised association
- [ ] **D** The genetic defect responsible for this condition is located on the short arm of chromosome 16
- [ ] **E** End-stage renal failure occurs in 90% of such patients by the age of 50

79. A 32-year-old man presents with syncopal episodes. Clinical examination reveals a jerky pulse character and harsh ejection systolic murmur at the left sternal edge. Echocardiography is performed and shows asymmetrical septal hypertrophy. What are this man's syncopal episodes most likely to be caused by?

- [ ] **A** Atrial tachyarrhythmias
- [ ] **B** Bradyarrhythmias
- [ ] **C** Multifactorial left ventricular outflow-tract obstruction
- [ ] **D** Systolic anterior motion of the anterior mitral valve leaflet
- [ ] **E** Ventricular tachyarrhythmias

80. A 68-year-old woman presents with a two-day history of abdominal cramp and diarrhoea. She has had five to six bowel motions each day and has noted blood mixed with stools on the day of presentation. She feels nauseous, but has not vomited. The symptoms appear to be getting worse. She has been visiting her son and had her meals with her son's family at home for the past week, but reports that her granddaughter was admitted yesterday to the children's ward with similar symptoms. They have not been abroad recently. On examination, she is afebrile, but looks pale and in discomfort, pulse 106 bpm, blood pressure 104/40 mmHg. There is diffuse but marked tenderness on abdominal examination, but no guarding, rigidity or rebound tenderness. Investigations: haemoglobin 10.2 g/dl, WCC 12.4 × 10⁹/l, platelets: 104 × 10⁹ /l, MCV 98.0 fl, blood smear shows burr cells +, clotting profile is normal, urea 14 mmol/l, creatinine 218 μmol/l, sodium 144 mmol/l, potassium 5 mmol/l, total bilirubin 24 μmol/l, albumin 34 g/l, ALT 56 U/L, ALP 113 U/l, stool microscopy white blood cells + +, red blood cells + + +. Which one of the following is the most important next step in the management of this patient?

- [ ] **A** Request stool sample to be screened for *Escherichia coli* O157:H7
- [ ] **B** Request an urgent mesenteric angiogram
- [ ] **C** Start on intravenous broad-spectrum antibiotics covering enteric organisms
- [ ] **D** Start on intravenous hydrocortisone
- [ ] **E** Arrange for haemodialysis

81. **Drug clearance is one of the major determinants of steady-state plasma concentrations. Which one of the following best describes the pattern of zero-order (non-linear) elimination kinetics?**

    ☐ **A** Complete inhibition of hepatic enzymes in response to increased drug doses

    ☐ **B** Drug concentrations do not increase despite increases in the administered dose

    ☐ **C** Drug concentrations rise in proportion to increases in the administered dose

    ☐ **D** Saturation of protein binding sites associated with increased drug doses results in significantly increased drug clearance

    ☐ **E** The rate of elimination does not increase in response to increased drug doses due to saturation of metabolising enzymes

82. **A 35-year-old army officer presents to hospital with episodes of dizziness and occasional blackouts. ECG examination reveals complete heart block. It is also noticed that he is suffering from a left third nerve palsy. He has previously been completely fit, and has recently returned from training exercises in Germany. While abroad, he describes a period of flu-like symptoms associated with a rash which started as a small red spot and expanded outwards into a large red circle. What is the rash most likely to have been?**

    ☐ **A** Erythema multiforme
    ☐ **B** Erythema chronicum migrans
    ☐ **C** Erythema annulare centrifugum
    ☐ **D** Erythema gyratum repens
    ☐ **E** Erythema ab igne

83. A 50-year-old woman with a body mass index of 35 kg/m² is found to have diabetes. After 12 weeks, it is clear that diet alone will not achieve adequate glycaemic control. She has no other past medical history of note. Which one of the following would be the treatment of choice?

☐ **A** Gliclazide
☐ **B** Metformin
☐ **C** Glibenclamide
☐ **D** Insulin
☐ **E** Rosiglitazone

84. A 56-year-old, poorly controlled, insulin-dependent diabetic complains of horizontal diplopia. Diplopia is maximal on left gaze, and covering the left eye leads to disappearance of the outer image. Which nerve is most likely to be affected?

☐ **A** Right abducens
☐ **B** Left abducens
☐ **C** Right oculomotor
☐ **D** Left oculomotor
☐ **E** Left trochlear

85. A 32-year-old man presents to the Accident and Emergency Department with a history of vomiting 'coffee grounds' earlier in the day. He was well until three days previously when he noticed that he had developed extensive bruising on his legs. He smokes 20 cigarettes per day and ingests 30 units of alcohol per week. On examination he is pale and has extensive bruising on his arms and legs. He has some epigastric tenderness. Laboratory investigations reveal: haemoglobin 5.5 g/dl, WCC 1.5 × 10⁹/l, neutrophils 0.3 × 10⁹/l, lymphocytes 1.2 × 10⁹/l with occasional atypical cells, possibly blasts, on the film, platelets 2 × 10⁹/l, prothrombin time 18 s (normal range 12–17 s), APTT 44 s (normal range 24–38 s), thrombin time 21 s (normal range 14–22 s), fibrinogen 0.5 g/l (normal range 2–5 g/l) and fibrin degradation products 140 µg/ml (normal range < 10 µg/ml). Which one of the following is the most likely underlying diagnosis?

- [ ] **A** Acute lymphoblastic leukaemia
- [ ] **B** Alcohol-induced gastritis
- [ ] **C** Disseminated intravascular coagulation due to carcinoma of the stomach
- [ ] **D** Aplastic anaemia
- [ ] **E** Acute promyelocytic leukaemia

86. A 24-year-old man has been admitted for observation following an episode of palpitations and cardiac arrhythmia. Two days after admission, nursing staff report that the patient is orientated but behaving strangely and at times talks to himself. You believe he is acutely psychotic and want to exclude a drug-induced psychosis. A positive urine screen to which one of the following drugs would NOT suggest that illicit drugs may be contributing to his psychosis?

- [ ] **A** Amphetamine
- [ ] **B** Cannabis
- [ ] **C** Cocaine
- [ ] **D** Heroin
- [ ] **E** Phencyclidine

87. A 49-year-old man is brought to the Accident and Emergency Department following an episode of acute shortness of breath. He has been put on oxygen via a low-flow face mask (with side holes) with the oxygen flow rate set at 2 l/min. His breathing has improved and his respiratory rate has returned to normal. What is the approximate fractional inspired oxygen concentration (FiO_2)?

- ☐ **A** 24%
- ☐ **B** 28%
- ☐ **C** 35%
- ☐ **D** 40%
- ☐ **E** 50%

88. A 32-year-old man presents with a four-month history of back pain. The pain is worse in the morning and after sitting watching TV. Plain X-ray of the spine/pelvis shows evidence of sacroiliitis. Each of the following clinical features might be identified on clinical examination of this patient, except:

- ☐ **A** Keratoderma blennorrhagica
- ☐ **B** Rheumatoid nodule
- ☐ **C** Onycholysis
- ☐ **D** Uveitis
- ☐ **E** Urethritis

89. Three days after arriving in the UK from Sri Lanka, a 45-year-old woman develops a fever of 39 °C, headache and severe myalgia. Examination is unremarkable apart from a 15-mmHg postural drop in systolic blood pressure and petechiae on the lower legs. A single thick blood film is negative for malarial parasites. The white blood cell count is at the lower limit of normal and the platelet count is 35×10^9/l. What is the most likely diagnosis?

- ☐ **A** *Plasmodium vivax* malaria
- ☐ **B** *Plasmodium falciparum* malaria
- ☐ **C** *Salmonella typhi*
- ☐ **D** *Rickettsia typhi*
- ☐ **E** Dengue fever

90. An 18-year-old man is sent for review at Cardiology Outpatients after a heart murmur was detected at a routine medical check-up in Occupational Health. He denies having any cardiac symptoms. Examination findings are: sinus rhythm with an ejection systolic murmur and fixed splitting of the second heart sound. His ECG shows right axis deviation of the QRS complex and large P waves. Which one of the following is the correct diagnosis?

- ☐ **A** Fallot's tetralogy
- ☐ **B** Ostium primum atrial septal defect
- ☐ **C** Ostium secundum atrial septal defect
- ☐ **D** Patent foramen ovale
- ☐ **E** Small ventricular septal defect

91. A 32-year-old woman with chronic asthma has been treated with theophylline for several years. Her General Practitioner had recently prescribed an additional treatment for a new illness. Shortly afterwards, she complained of palpitations, serum theophylline concentrations were found to be above the normal therapeutic range, and theophylline toxicity is suspected. Which one of the following drugs is most likely to have been responsible?

- ☐ **A** Aspirin
- ☐ **B** Carbimazole
- ☐ **C** Erythromycin
- ☐ **D** Oral contraceptive pill
- ☐ **E** Sertraline

92. A 42-year-old man received a cadaveric renal transplant seven years ago. His primary disease was chronic pyelonephritis due to vesico-ureteric reflux. The postoperative course was uneventful with immediate graft function and a creatinine at discharge of 123 μmol/l. Maintenance immunosuppression was ciclosporin 200 mg bd and prednisolone 7.5 mg daily. He also took atenolol 50 mg once daily and simvastatin 20 mg once a day. Transplant function was stable until two years ago when the plasma creatinine began to rise, reaching a present level of 186 μmol/l. Blood pressure remains well controlled at 136/72 mmHg. Transplant biopsy demonstrated normal glomeruli with interstitial fibrosis and tubular dropout. Which cytokine is most likely to be shown on immunostaining in both glomeruli and the interstitium?

☐ A IL-4
☐ B IL-8
☐ C IFN-γ
☐ D TGF-β
☐ E TNF-α

93. A 16-year-old boy presents with a six-week history of a non-itchy rash affecting his chest, back and upper arms. He is otherwise well. On examination, there are a large number of erythematous/brownish macules present on his trunk and arms, which have a fine scale. On screening with Wood's light, the lesions fluoresce pale yellow. He is treated with topical selenium sulphide with full clearance of the rash. What is the most likely diagnosis?

☐ A Pityriasis versicolor
☐ B Pityriasis rosea
☐ C Guttate psoriasis
☐ D Cutaneous larva migrans
☐ E Scabies

94. A 50-year-old Asian lady is feeling weak, with generalised aches and pains. On examination, she is unable to get up from a chair without using her arms. Blood results show: corrected calcium 2.20 mmol/l (normal range 2.25–2.70 mmol/l), alkaline phosphatase 150 U/l (normal range 20–120 U/l). Which one of the following is the most likely diagnosis?

☐ **A** Osteomalacia
☐ **B** Primary hypoparathyroidism
☐ **C** Polymyalgia rheumatica
☐ **D** Paget's disease of bone
☐ **E** Polymyositis

95. A 70-year-old lady presents with anorexia of three weeks' duration. She has noticed dark urine for the past two weeks. She has a dull ache in the right upper abdomen, but denies any fever, rigor or itching. She has been diagnosed with hypothyroidism for six years, treated with thyroxine 100 μg daily; hypercholesterolaemia, for which she has taken simvastatin 20–40 mg daily for five years; and hypertension for 18 months, for which she has been on amlodipine 10 mg daily. She has had low backache for the past year and has been diagnosed with Paget's disease, treated with diclofenac sodium 50 mg twice a day for the past 4½ months. She drinks about six glasses of wine per week and has not travelled abroad recently. On examination she is jaundiced, but no other signs suggestive of chronic liver disease are found. Abdominal examination is normal. Investigations: total bilirubin 112 μmol/l, albumin 40 g/l, ALT 980 U/l, ALP 880 U/l, IgG 11.5 g/l, IgA 1.4 g/l, IgM 1.2 g/l, anti-nuclear antibody positive at 1/80, thyroid microsomal antibody positive at 1/800, anti-smooth muscle antibody negative, anti-liver-kidney-microsomal antibody negative, serology for hepatitis A, B and C virus negative. Ultrasound examination of her abdomen shows normal echotexture of the liver with no intrahepatic duct dilatation. The gallbladder, spleen and kidneys are normal, and the pancreas is obscured by bowel gas. Which one of the following is true regarding the management of this patient?

☐ **A** Validity of self-reporting of alcohol intake should be questioned as the pattern of liver injury suggests acute alcoholic hepatitis
☐ **B** ERCP is indicated to exclude pancreatic cancer
☐ **C** Diclofenac should be withdrawn immediately
☐ **D** Treatment with prednisolone should be started immediately
☐ **E** The degree of ALT elevation indicates a poor prognosis

96. A 70-year-old woman presents with tiredness and easy bruising and frequent infections. On examination she has a few bruises on her legs and a septic lesion on her right hand. Her haemoglobin is 6.3 g/dl, MCV 105 fl, WCC 4.5 × 10⁹/l with neutrophils of 0.9 × 10⁹/l, lymphocytes 3.3 × 10⁹/l and monocytes 0.3 × 10⁹/l, platelets 52 × 10⁹/l and reticulocytes 75 × 10⁹/l (normal range 50–100 × 10⁹/l). Which one of the following is the most likely haematological diagnosis?

- [ ] **A** Vitamin B_{12} deficiency
- [ ] **B** Myelodysplastic syndrome
- [ ] **C** Acute myeloid leukaemia
- [ ] **D** Folic acid deficiency
- [ ] **E** Chronic myelomonocytic leukaemia

97. A 63-year-old man presents with reduced visual acuity in the left eye. This eye sees 6/36 and fundoscopy reveals extensive retinal haemorrhages and cotton wool spots. The right eye sees 6/9 and the fundal examination is normal. What is the most likely diagnosis?

- [ ] **A** Grade 2 hypertensive retinopathy
- [ ] **B** Background diabetic retinopathy
- [ ] **C** Preproliferative diabetic retinopathy
- [ ] **D** Central retinal vein occlusion
- [ ] **E** Grade 3 hypertensive retinopathy

98. A 26-year-old patient describes the distressing feeling that people around her appear lifeless and the environment seems very flat. Which one of the following best describes her experience?

- [ ] **A** Depersonalisation
- [ ] **B** Derealisation
- [ ] **C** *Jamais vu*
- [ ] **D** Delusional mood
- [ ] **E** 'Free-floating' anxiety

99. A 38-year-old woman weighing 100 kg, and 170 cm tall, presents with frontal headache and bilateral visual disturbance. On examination, her visual acuity is 6/18 bilaterally, adduction of the right eye is impaired and there is bilateral papilloedema on fundoscopy. An urgent CT scan of the head is normal. What is the most likely diagnosis?

☐ A Sagittal sinus thrombosis
☐ B Hypoparathyroidism
☐ C Frontal astrocytoma
☐ D Normal-pressure hydrocephalus
☐ E Benign intracranial hypertension

100. A 69-year-old man is referred for a cardiopulmonary exercise test because of unexplained episodes of breathlessness. His FEV_1 is 2.1 litres and FVC 2.9 litres. The results are shown below:

	Actual	Predicted	% Predicted
VO_2max (l/min)	1.19	1.91	62
VEmax (l/min)	37.2	73.5	51
VO_2max	= maximum oxygen uptake		
VEmax	= maximum ventilation		

He reaches a peak heart rate of 142 bpm and his oxygen saturation (SaO_2) drops from a baseline of 96% on air (at rest) to 89% at peak exercise. Which one of the following is the most likely explanation for these findings?

☐ A Normal results
☐ B Cardiac disease
☐ C Pulmonary vascular disease
☐ D Restrictive lung disease
☐ E Obstructive lung disease

101. A 28-year-old teacher is admitted to hospital with a three-week history of exhaustion, dyspnoea, fever and chills, and 15–20 pounds of weight loss. She is known to have SLE and was maintained on steroids and azathioprine. Her chest radiograph showed bilateral lower lobe infiltrates. Each of the following tests would support the diagnosis of SLE pneumonitis rather than bronchopneumonia, except:

  ☐ **A** High titres of anti-dsDNA
  ☐ **B** Elevated CRP concentration
  ☐ **C** High ESR levels
  ☐ **D** Low C3/C4 complement levels
  ☐ **E** Red blood cell casts in urine sediment

102. A positive correlation is found between weight and systolic blood pressure amongst a group of ten-year-old children ($r=0.7$, 95% CI (0.52 to 0.88), $P=0.0004$). What is the most appropriate conclusion to be drawn from this correlation?

  ☐ **A** Before weight loss can occur, systolic blood pressure must be lowered
  ☐ **B** Those with high systolic blood pressures are more likely to be obese
  ☐ **C** There is a significant tendency for heavier ten-year-olds to have higher systolic blood pressures
  ☐ **D** Weight affects systolic blood pressure
  ☐ **E** There is a non-significant tendency for heavier ten-year-olds to have higher systolic blood pressures

103. A 73-year-old woman with a history of multiple pulmonary emboli complains to her GP of increasing shortness of breath on exertion. She denies having any orthopnoea or cough. The GP suspects secondary pulmonary hypertension has developed and asks you to see her urgently in Outpatients. What findings on auscultation would be most likely to support this diagnosis?

  ☐ **A** Fixed splitting of the second heart sound
  ☐ **B** Gallop rhythm
  ☐ **C** Widely split second heart sound
  ☐ **D** Loud, early pulmonary second sound
  ☐ **E** Mid-systolic click

104. Which one of the following pharmacokinetic factors is NOT significantly altered by renal impairment?

☐ **A** Absorption from the gastrointestinal tract
☐ **B** Bioavailability following intravenous administration
☐ **C** Drug distribution
☐ **D** Hepatic metabolism
☐ **E** Renal tubular drug secretion

105. A 20-year-old man arrived in the UK from East Africa a month ago. He gives a three-month history of marked weight loss and daily fever with night sweats. Examination reveals an ill, wasted man with massive splenomegaly. Investigations confirm the suspected clinical diagnosis. What is the most appropriate treatment?

☐ **A** Zidovudine, lamivudine, lopinavir and ritonavir
☐ **B** Rifampicin, isoniazid, pyrazinamide and ethambutol
☐ **C** Quinine and doxycycline
☐ **D** Intravenous amphotericin
☐ **E** Praziquantel

106. A 72-year-old lady presents with a six-week history of an itchy urticaria-like rash on her arms and legs. She then develops large fluid-filled blisters on her limbs and central abdomen. The blisters remain intact for two or three days before rupturing. Her mucosal membranes are clear. A skin biopsy shows a subepidermal blister with eosinophils, and immunofluorescence demonstrates linear IgG and C3 deposition at the basement membrane. What is the most likely diagnosis?

☐ **A** Pemphigoid gestationis
☐ **B** Pemphigus vulgaris
☐ **C** Bullous pemphigoid
☐ **D** Cicatricial pemphigoid
☐ **E** Dermatitis herpetiformis

107. A 24-year-old woman is admitted for a parathyroidectomy. The Surgical House Officer takes a detailed history, and notes on review of systems that the patient has had secondary amenorrhoea for three years, and that her mother also had a parathyroidectomy operation at the age of 40. Regarding the patient's secondary amenorrhoea, which one of the following tests is the most important?

- [ ] A Thyroid function tests
- [ ] B Serum progesterone
- [ ] C Serum gonadotrophins (LH and FSH)
- [ ] D Serum prolactin
- [ ] E Serum oestrogen

108. A 34-year-old woman consults her GP complaining of painful, stiff hands. A history of Raynaud's phenomenon is elicited. She is found to have a blood pressure of 174/98 mmHg and haematuria and proteinuria on dipstick urine testing. Investigations demonstrate: creatinine 134 μmol/l, haemoglobin 11.8 g/dl, CRP 4 mg/l, ESR 68 mm/h, ANA positive at 1/320. What is renal biopsy most likely to show?

- [ ] A Proliferative glomerulonephritis with subendothelial deposits
- [ ] B Proliferative glomerulonephritis with mesangial IgA staining
- [ ] C Necrotising glomerulonephritis with cellular crescent formation
- [ ] D Proliferative glomerulonephritis with spikes on silver staining
- [ ] E Proliferative glomerulonephritis with ' full house' immunostaining

109. Two Caucasian siblings attend Haematology regularly for transfusion. They have a lifelong history of anaemia and had their spleens removed at two and three years of age respectively. There is no previous family history of anaemia. A typical blood count pre-transfusion is as follows: haemoglobin 7.2 g/dl, MCV 105 fl, WCC 6.2 × 10⁹/l with a normal differential, platelets 252 × 10⁹/l and reticulocytes 230 x 10⁹/l (normal range 50–100 × 10⁹/l). Blood film shows post-splenectomy changes and 'prickle' or 'sputnik' cells. Which one of the following is the most likely cause of their anaemia?

- [ ] A Thalassaemia intermedia
- [ ] B Autoimmune haemolytic anaemia
- [ ] C Pyruvate kinase deficiency
- [ ] D Hereditary spherocytosis
- [ ] E G6PD deficiency

110. A 70-year-old woman was admitted with an infective exacerbation of chronic obstructive airways disease. She was treated with regular nebulised bronchodilators, oral prednisolone 30 mg daily and intravenous cefuroxime 750 mg three times a day. Her respiratory symptoms improved over the next five days. Six days after her admission she developed frequent loose motions, ten times a day, associated with lower abdominal discomfort, urgency and occasional incontinence. There has been no blood in the stools. Abdominal examination reveals increased bowel sounds and no other abnormalities. Investigations show: haemoglobin 15.9 g/dl, WCC 11.5 × 10⁹/l, platelets 460 × 10⁹/l, stool microscopy showing white blood cells + +. Which one of the following is most likely to be correct regarding antibiotic-associated colitis?

- [ ] A *Clostridium difficile* causes colitis by direct invasion of bowel mucosa
- [ ] B Detection of *C. difficile* toxin in the stool sample is diagnostic
- [ ] C Positive stool culture is the most specific test for the diagnosis
- [ ] D Rigid sigmoidoscopy is the most sensitive test as pseudomembranes are seen in the rectum in over 90% of cases
- [ ] E Vancomycin is the drug of first choice and should be started early to be effective

111. A 52-year-old man presents with a right-sided inferonasal quadrantanopia.
     Which of the following is true?

☐ **A** The lesion is in the region of the optic chiasm
☐ **B** The lesion is in the right parietal lobe
☐ **C** The lesion is in the left parietal lobe
☐ **D** The lesion is in the right temporal lobe
☐ **E** A carotid Doppler should be performed

112. A 36-year-old woman has presented with her fourth overdose in the last 12 months. You believe it is important this lady gets appropriate help to reduce the future risk of self-harm. In trying to discover whether this lady has a mental illness or a personality disorder, which one of the following from her history would most lead you to conclude the latter?

☐ **A** A long history of deliberate self-harm when younger
☐ **B** Continuous history of adverse effects on society
☐ **C** Experiencing the hearing of voices inside her head
☐ **D** Poor coping mechanisms from her mid-twenties onwards
☐ **E** The patient is superficially charming

113. A 72-year-old man presents with acute onset of right-sided incoordination. On examination he has a right Horner's syndrome and loss of sensation to pinprick on the left side of his face. Which artery is most likely to have been occluded?

☐ **A** Vertebral artery
☐ **B** Superior cerebellar artery
☐ **C** Posterior cerebral artery
☐ **D** Basilar artery
☐ **E** Posterior inferior cerebellar artery

114. A 29-year-old woman with asthma comes to the clinic with poorly controlled symptoms of cough, wheeze and breathlessness. Her current treatment includes beclometasone dipropionate 800 μg/day using a spacer and salbutamol as required. You check her inhaler technique, which is very good. What would your next management step be?

- ☐ **A** One week of oral prednisolone
- ☐ **B** Add oral theophylline
- ☐ **C** Add oral leukotriene receptor antagonist
- ☐ **D** Add a long-acting β$_2$-agonist
- ☐ **E** Increase the dose of inhaled steroids

115. A 30-year-old man who has just been released from prison in eastern Europe arrives in the UK. In prison over the past two years he has, intermittently, had different drug regimes of one or two drugs at a time for pulmonary TB. He has extensive cavitation on his chest X-ray and sputum is smear-positive for AAFB. What is the most appropriate course of action?

- ☐ **A** Respiratory isolation, continuing for two weeks from the start of TB therapy
- ☐ **B** Treatment with standard quadruple anti-TB therapy until sensitivities are known
- ☐ **C** Polymerase chain reaction (PCR) for resistance genes to all first-line drugs
- ☐ **D** Offer HIV testing
- ☐ **E** Give close contacts isoniazid prophylaxis

116. A 52-year-old diabetic woman with a history of exertional chest pain presents with retrosternal chest pain associated with T-wave inversion in the chest leads. Her troponin I is five times the upper limit of normal the following morning. Which single investigation will provide most diagnostic information?

- ☐ **A** Cardiac catheterisation
- ☐ **B** Echocardiography
- ☐ **C** Exercise stress testing
- ☐ **D** Holter monitoring (24-hour ECG)
- ☐ **E** Radionuclide cardiac perfusion scanning

117. A 35-year-old man presents with a rash on his feet. There is a recent history of a diarrhoeal episode. He also now complains of sore joints and gritty, red eyes. On examination of his feet, there are multiple red papules with slight scaling, pustules and areas of hyperkeratosis. What is this skin eruption most likely to represent?

- [ ] **A** Pustular psoriasis
- [ ] **B** Tinea pedis
- [ ] **C** Keratoderma blennorrhagica
- [ ] **D** Pompholyx
- [ ] **E** Acanthosis nigricans

118. A patient with type 1 diabetes mellitus diagnosed 11 years previously is found to have albuminuria on routine screening. He had laser treatment for proliferative retinopathy four years ago. Plasma creatinine is 104 μmol/l, Hb A_{1c} 8.3% and albumin excretion 310 mg/24 h. Which of the following would be shown on renal biopsy?

- [ ] **A** Kimmelstiel-Wilson lesions
- [ ] **B** Spikes on silver staining
- [ ] **C** Mesangial IgA deposition
- [ ] **D** Proliferative glomerulonephritis with 'full house' immunostaining
- [ ] **E** Foot process effacement on electron microscopy

119. A 60-year-old man is admitted with lobar pneumonia and a history of recent weight loss. He is tachycardic on admission. Thyroid function tests are checked. The results are as follows: TSH 0.1 mU/l (normal range 0.3–4 mU/l), FT4 8 pmol/l (normal range 10–24 pmol/l). Which one of the following is the most likely explanation of these results?

- [ ] **A** Primary hyperthyroidism
- [ ] **B** Secondary hyperthyroidism
- [ ] **C** Sick euthyroid syndrome
- [ ] **D** Primary hypothyroidism
- [ ] **E** Secondary hypothyroidism

120. A 58-year-old man has a three-month history of low back pain. He presents to the Accident and Emergency Department with a two-day history of increasing confusion and blurred vision. On examination he is pale and tender over his lumbar spine. His Glasgow Coma Scale score is 11 and he has retinal haemorrhages. His haemoglobin is 9.3 g/dl, MCV 102 fl, WCC 3.5×10^9/l with a normal differential, platelets 120×10^9/l, urea 10 mmol/l, Na$^+$ 139 mmol/l, K$^+$ 4.6 mmol/l, creatinine 180 umol/l, total protein 88 g/l, albumin 24 g/l, and viscosity 8.2 cP (normal range 1.5–1.72 cP). Skeletal survey shows widespread lytic lesions. Which one of the following is the most important immediate management of this patient's condition?

- ☐ **A** Transfusion of packed cells
- ☐ **B** Urgent plasmapheresis
- ☐ **C** Immediate chemotherapy
- ☐ **D** Intravenous fluids
- ☐ **E** Prednisolone

121. A 43-year-old woman with a previous diagnosis of autoimmune hepatitis and cirrhosis is referred with abdominal distension and weight gain. On examination she weighs 108 kg and has bilateral pitting ankle oedema. She is not jaundiced. Abdominal distension is noted and shifting dullness could be elicited. Which one of the following is the most important mechanism leading to the development of fluid retention in this patient?

- ☐ **A** Hypoalbuminaemia
- ☐ **B** Portal hypertension
- ☐ **C** Lymphatic obstruction due to regenerative nodules
- ☐ **D** Obstruction of the inferior vena cava by regenerative nodules
- ☐ **E** Increased sodium absorption in the renal tubules

122. A 68-year-old woman has been referred to you with a history of progressive intellectual deterioration. As part of your assessment you perform a cognitive examination and find that her deficits appear to indicate parietal lobe dysfunction. Which one of the following is least consistent with such a diagnosis?

- [ ] **A** Anosognosia
- [ ] **B** Autotopagnosia
- [ ] **C** Structional apraxia
- [ ] **D** Prosopagnosia
- [ ] **E** Right–left disorientation

123. A 67-year-old man with chronic obstructive pulmonary disease is brought to the Accident and Emergency Department with acute shortness of breath and a cough productive of green sputum. His last FEV$_1$ in the clinic three months ago, when he was well, was 1.2 litres. On examination he has coarse inspiratory crackles at the right base and a fever of 38.9 °C. His chest X-ray shows some shadowing in the right lower zone and arterial blood gases on 24% oxygen show: pH 7.38, PaCO$_2$ 8.9 kPa, PaO$_2$ 6.1 kPa, bicarbonate 36 mmol/l. Which one of the following would be your next management step?

- [ ] **A** Increase the inspired oxygen
- [ ] **B** Intravenous doxapram
- [ ] **C** Continuous positive airways pressure (CPAP)
- [ ] **D** Intubation and mechanical ventilation
- [ ] **E** Bi-level positive airways pressure (BiPAP)

124. A 44-year-old man presents with a four-day history of back pain, deteriorating gait, and paraesthesiae in both hands and feet. On examination there is lower limb weakness bilaterally, areflexia and urinary retention. What is the most likely diagnosis?

- [ ] **A** Acute poliomyelitis
- [ ] **B** Brown-Séquard syndrome
- [ ] **C** Guillain-Barré syndrome
- [ ] **D** Lumbar canal stenosis
- [ ] **E** Subacute combined degeneration of the cord

125. A 77-year-old man presents with persistent headache and progressive deafness. On examination he has frontal bossing of the forehead and conductive deafness, more severe in the right ear. The alkaline phosphatase was significantly raised at 870 U/l. At this point in the patient's evaluation, which one of the following tests is MOST appropriate?

- [ ] **A** Magnetic resonance imaging (MRI) of the skull
- [ ] **B** Isotope bone scan
- [ ] **C** Plain X-ray of the skull
- [ ] **D** Bone mineral densitometry
- [ ] **E** Ultrasound examination of the liver

126. A patient is brought to the emergency department feeling dizzy and nauseous. This is the first episode he has experienced and he has no other medical history or regular medication. Blood pressure is 110/60 mmHg and the radial pulse rate is 180 bpm. Examination is otherwise unremarkable. An ECG shows broad-complex tachycardia, rate 180 bpm. There are no previous ECGs for comparison. What ECG findings would best support a ventricular origin for this tachycardia?

- [ ] **A** Concordance in the chest leads
- [ ] **B** Capture and fusion beats
- [ ] **C** Left bundle pattern
- [ ] **D** Right bundle pattern
- [ ] **E** QRS duration over 180 ms

127. A 50-year-old man, initially thought to have primary hypothyroidism, is subsequently found to have panhypopituitarism. Which one of the following treatments should be started first?

- [ ] **A** Thyroxine
- [ ] **B** Testosterone
- [ ] **C** Fludrocortisone
- [ ] **D** Growth hormone
- [ ] **E** Hydrocortisone

128. A newly diagnosed 27-year-old HIV-positive woman is admitted with a CD4 count of 2 cells/μl. *Mycobacterium avium-intracellulare* is grown from blood cultures and she is treated with appropriate antibiotics. She is also started on highly active antiretroviral therapy at the same time. Four weeks later she is admitted with severe abdominal pain and fevers. Computed tomography scan of the abdomen shows marked, widespread para-aortic lymphadenopathy. What is the most likely diagnosis?

☐ A Lymphoma
☐ B Immune reconstitution illness
☐ C Extra-pulmonary *Pneumocystis jiroveci (carinii)*
☐ D Cytomegalovirus
☐ E Cryptococcosis

129. A 35-year-old man presents to the Accident and Emergency Department with bruising and laceration to his head following involvement in a fight. He says that he has a history of haemophilia B. On examination he has several superficial lacerations and extensive bruising. His level of consciousness is not impaired. Skull X-ray does not show any abnormality. Which one of the following represents the most important immediate management of his condition?

☐ A Infusion of factor VIII concentrate
☐ B Infusion of fresh frozen plasma
☐ C Infusion of cryoprecipitate
☐ D Intramuscular pethidine
☐ E Infusion of factor IX concentrate

130. A 46-year-old man has an anterior cruciate ligament repair under general anaesthetic. Routine preoperative investigations, including dipstick urinalysis are unremarkable. He makes an uneventful recovery and is discharged home with indometacin. Two weeks later he presents to his GP with marked ankle oedema. His GP finds his blood pressure to be 128/76 mmHg. Dipstick urinalysis reveals protein + + + but no haematuria. Plasma creatinine is normal. What is the most likely diagnosis?

- [ ] **A** Acute tubular necrosis
- [ ] **B** Interstitial nephritis
- [ ] **C** Lupus nephritis
- [ ] **D** Membranous nephropathy
- [ ] **E** Minimal change nephropathy

131. A 51-year-old man comes to the clinic with long-standing episodes of breathlessness. He has been followed-up at his local hospital for many years but wants a second opinion. When you review his multiple chest X-rays over the last five years you notice a pattern of flitting multifocal consolidation. Which of the following diagnoses is the least likely?

- [ ] **A** Cryptogenic organising pneumonia
- [ ] **B** Langerhans cell histiocytosis
- [ ] **C** Allergic bronchopulmonary aspergillosis
- [ ] **D** Eosinophilic pneumonia
- [ ] **E** Sarcoidosis

132. A 32-year-old white man presents with gradual onset of central colicky abdominal pain over a period of 5 weeks' associated with diarrhoea, loss of weight and anorexia. Stool cultures were negative. On examination he is unwell with a temperature of 37.8 °C and pulse 118 bpm. He has multiple aphthoid ulcers in the mouth and is tender in the right iliac fossa. Investigations reveal: haemoglobin 10.1 g/dl, WCC 12.8 × 10⁹/l, platelets 690 × 10⁹/l, vitamin B₁₂, folate and iron studies within the normal range. CRP was 99 mg/l; LFTs, urea and electrolytes normal. Which one of the following is true with regards to the clinical scenario?

☐ A Laparotomy is indicated as the likely diagnosis is acute appendicitis

☐ B Negative stool culture excludes *Yersinia* enterocolitis

☐ C Small bowel contrast studies should be performed to look for ileal Crohn's disease

☐ D Ulceration of the small bowel is the commonest gastrointestinal manifestation of Behçet's disease

☐ E Colonoscopy is the investigation of choice as abdominal pain is typical of ulcerative colitis

133. A 65-year-old woman reports difficulty walking. She can walk for one block, but pain in both knees forces her to stop and sit, which relieves the pain. Her doctor thought she had osteoarthritis of the knee and he ordered radiographs of the knee. Which one of the following is NOT a characteristic radiographic finding of osteoarthritis?

☐ A Osteophytes
☐ B Asymmetrical joint-space narrowing
☐ C Subchondral cysts
☐ D Marginal erosions
☐ E Subchondral bone sclerosis

134. **A 64-year-old smoker presents to the Accident and Emergency Department with sudden onset of flaccid weakness of both legs and urinary incontinence, associated with thoracic back pain. On examination there is bilateral leg weakness, decreased sensation to pinprick below T7, but preserved joint-position sense in the lower limbs. What is the most likely diagnosis?**

☐ **A** Anterior spinal artery occlusion
☐ **B** Acute transverse myelitis
☐ **C** Intramedullary glioma
☐ **D** Vertebral collapse secondary to metastasis
☐ **E** Syringomyelia

135. **A 40-year-old lorry driver with a strong family history of ischaemic heart disease presents with chest pain and ST elevation in leads II, AVF and III. He is treated with streptokinase and makes a good recovery. By day 5 he is established on aspirin, atenolol, ramipril and simvastatin. You speak to him about lifestyle modifications and raise the subject of driving. He states that he wishes to resume his lorry-driving career. What is the most appropriate advice to give him?**

☐ **A** He should inform the DVLA and will be banned from LGV driving for life but may resume driving a private vehicle after one month
☐ **B** He may resume driving a private motor car after one month and an LGV after six months if symptom-free
☐ **C** He should inform the DVLA and may resume driving a private vehicle after one month if passed fit but will be required to undergo coronary angiography to regain his LGV licence
☐ **D** He should inform the DVLA and may resume driving a private vehicle after one month if passed fit but will be required to complete three stages of the Bruce protocol off anti-anginals and without evidence of ischaemia to regain LGV entitlement
☐ **E** He should inform the DVLA who will withdraw all licences but may consider re-licensing for private motor car and LGV after six months

136. A randomised controlled trial of a new therapy for hypertension shows a statistically significant difference (P=0.0012) between treatment and placebo. The group which received the new therapy tended to have a lower body mass index (BMI), and this may have contributed to the difference observed in blood pressure at the end of the study. Which one of the following would be the most appropriate interpretation/action?

- [ ] A All those with BMI > 30 should be excluded and the analysis re-done
- [ ] B The new therapy is significantly better, no further action need be taken, and it should be introduced as standard
- [ ] C Since the trial is randomised, the result must be correct and differences in BMI can be ignored
- [ ] D The data should be re-analysed for low and high BMI values
- [ ] E BMI may be a confounder – it should be corrected for in the analysis

137. A 41-year-old man is receiving erythromycin for suspected prostatitis. Which one of the following is not a recognised adverse effect of erythromycin antibiotic treatment?

- [ ] A Cholestatic jaundice
- [ ] B Hepatic enzyme inhibition
- [ ] C Increased small bowel propulsion
- [ ] D Prolongation of the QT interval
- [ ] E Stevens-Johnson syndrome

138. A 45-year-old man presents with erythroderma. He has a long history of chronic plaque psoriasis which has been well controlled with topical calcipotriol and emollients. He has never previously required admission to hospital for his psoriasis. However, he is now pyrexial, dehydrated and tachycardic. He had been started on a new medication six weeks previously by his GP, following which his psoriasis became unstable. Which one of the following drugs is the most likely cause?

- [ ] A Furosemide (frusemide)
- [ ] B Atenolol
- [ ] C Aspirin
- [ ] D Ibuprofen
- [ ] E Omeprazole

139. A previously well 50-year-old man is found to have endocarditis of his native, normal mitral valve. A fully sensitive *Streptococcus bovis* is subsequently isolated from multiple blood cultures. The vegetation is small, there is no cardiac failure and within a week of starting therapy he is afebrile and the CRP is normal. Which one of the following management plans would be LEAST appropriate?

- [ ] A Start treatment with meropenem and gentamicin prior to identification of the organism
- [ ] B Perform barium enema and/or colonoscopy
- [ ] C Continue treatment for one week more, then stop
- [ ] D Advise future prophylaxis for dental procedures
- [ ] E Refer to cardiac surgeons if patient suffers repeated embolic phenomena

140. A 23-year-old woman presents with marked swelling of the ankles following a mild upper respiratory tract infection. Dipstick testing of urine demonstrates protein +++ with no haematuria. Investigations show: plasma creatinine 68 μmol/l, albumin 23 g/dl, cholesterol 8.9 mmol/l urinary protein excretion 12g/24 h. A renal biopsy is performed which confirms minimal change glomerulopathy. She is commenced on prednisolone 60 mg/day and simvastatin. Seven days later, at a routine clinic visit, dipstick testing demonstrates protein +++ and blood ++. She has had some mild loin pain. Plasma creatinine is now 106 μmol/l. What is the most likely complication to have occurred?

- [ ] A Renal vein thrombosis
- [ ] B Interstitial nephritis secondary to simvastatin
- [ ] C Obstruction secondary to a sloughed papilla
- [ ] D Perinephric haemorrhage secondary to renal biopsy
- [ ] E Acute crescentic change of minimal change nephropathy

141. A plump 35-year-old lady with type 2 diabetes informs her GP that she is eight weeks pregnant. Her diabetes is currently treated with metformin and gliclazide. A recent Hb A_{1c} was 9%. Her GP gives her plenty of advice regarding her diabetes during her pregnancy. Which would you prioritise?

☐ A She should always have easy access to oral glucose
☐ B She should be more strict with her diet
☐ C She should be converted from tablets to insulin therapy
☐ D She should monitor her BMs more often
☐ E She should have her eyes checked

142. A 55-year-old man presents with a three-week history of myalgia and headache and a five-day history of jaundice. His past history includes depression for which he takes fluoxetine. He is brought to the hospital by his neighbours as he has been seen wandering in the front garden shouting at the passers-by. On examination he appears drowsy and confused, and is jaundiced. Investigations show: total bilirubin 135 μmol/l, albumin 44 g/l, ALT 4461 U/l, ALP 310 U/l, hepatitis-A IgM negative, HbsAg negative, prothrombin time 34 s, PT control 9.5 s, paracetamol level 43 mg/l. Which one of the following is the most appropriate statement regarding his prognosis?

☐ A High transaminases indicate a poor prognosis
☐ B Clinical and laboratory parameters indicate that the patient should be listed for liver transplantation
☐ C Patient's age is a factor predicting a poor prognosis without liver transplantation
☐ D Rapidity of development of encephalopathy (within one week of the onset of jaundice) is indicative of adverse outcome
☐ E Prognosis in acute hepatic failure is independent of the underlying cause

143. A 24-year-old woman is under investigation by a medical firm. She presented with a history of paleness, jaundice and dark urine in the morning. She was well until two months previously when she started to fell generally unwell. On examination she is anaemic and jaundiced. On investigation her haemoglobin is 8.4 g/dl, MCV 103 fl, WCC 3.8 × 10⁹/l with a normal differential, platelets 135 × 10⁹/l, reticulocytes 182 × 10⁹/l (normal range 50–100 × 10⁹/l), AST 22 U/l, ALT 23 U/l, ALP 95 U/l, bilirubin 44 μmol/l, LDH 1046 U/l. Which test is most likely to make the diagnosis?

- [ ] **A** Direct antiglobulin test
- [ ] **B** Ham's test
- [ ] **C** Bone marrow examination
- [ ] **D** Schumm's test
- [ ] **E** Urine examination

144. A 46-year-old woman with multiple sclerosis and asthma is attending for outpatient review. She appears to be clinically depressed. Which one of the following medications taken by this patient is least likely to produce depression?

- [ ] **A** Baclofen
- [ ] **B** Dantrolene
- [ ] **C** Diazepam
- [ ] **D** Interferon beta
- [ ] **E** Prednisolone

145. A 46-year-old woman presents with loss of sensation in her little finger. On examination she has weak dorsal interossei. What is the most likely site of her lesion?

- [ ] **A** Anterior interosseous nerve
- [ ] **B** Median nerve
- [ ] **C** Ulnar nerve
- [ ] **D** Radial nerve
- [ ] **E** Lower cord of brachial plexus

146. A 39-year-old Eastern European man has a bronchoscopy because he has right upper lobe consolidation with cavitation. He is not expectorating any sputum. Suspecting TB, you start him on anti-tuberculous chemotherapy and await the drug sensitivities. You are telephoned by the consultant microbiologist who tells you that your patient has multidrug resistant TB (MDRTB). Which one of the following anti-TB antibiotics is the patient resistant to?

- [ ] **A** Isoniazid, ethambutol and pyrazinamide
- [ ] **B** Rifampicin and isoniazid
- [ ] **C** Ethambutol and pyrazinamide
- [ ] **D** Isoniazid and streptomycin
- [ ] **E** Rifampicin, ethambutol and pyrazinamide

147. A 65-year-old man is referred for further management of gout. He had an episode of knee pain and swelling three weeks previously, and results of joint aspiration at that time were positive for uric acid crystals. Which one of the following findings would warrant uric acid-lowering therapy?

- [ ] **A** Creatinine level of 300 μmol/l (normal range 60–110 μmol/l)
- [ ] **B** Hypertension
- [ ] **C** Severe first attack of gout
- [ ] **D** Tophus of the ear
- [ ] **E** Uric acid level of 0.54 mmol/l (normal range 0–0.43 mmol/l)

148. A 23-year-old female school teacher develops a minor febrile illness which is followed a few days later by a reticular rash on the limbs and a swollen right knee. What is the most likely infecting agent?

- [ ] **A** Group A *Streptococcus*
- [ ] **B** Parvovirus B19
- [ ] **C** Rubella
- [ ] **D** Human herpesvirus 6 (HHV-6)
- [ ] **E** *Neisseria gonorrhoeae*

149. A 32-year-old man presents with marked ankle swelling. Blood pressure is 168/90 mmHg. Examination is otherwise unremarkable. Dipstick testing of the urine demonstrates protein +++ with no haematuria. Investigations demonstrate: plasma creatinine 164 μmol/l, albumin 16 g/dl and 24-hour urinary protein excretion of 8 g. Which one of the following statements is correct?

☐ **A** Barium enema should be performed to exclude carcinoma of the colon
☐ **B** The renal lesion is characterised by subendothelial deposits on biopsy
☐ **C** Male sex, hypertension and renal impairment at presentation are poor prognostic indicators
☐ **D** There is a recognised association with hepatitis C
☐ **E** The natural history of this condition is characterised by a rapid decline in renal function

150. A 78-year-old woman with paroxysmal atrial fibrillation is maintained on amiodarone. You see her for her routine follow-up: she is well but raises concerns about the long-term implications of amiodarone, as she has been told by a friend that it has a lot of side effects. She produces a long list of problems she has heard may be linked to the drug. Which of the following risks is most likely to be reversible on stopping amiodarone?

☐ **A** Alveolitis
☐ **B** Corneal opacification
☐ **C** Liver fibrosis
☐ **D** Peripheral neuropathy
☐ **E** Skin pigmentation

151. Which one of the following drugs is regarded as safe in a mother who is breastfeeding?

☐ **A** Aspirin
☐ **B** Carbimazole
☐ **C** Diazepam
☐ **D** Oxytetracycline
☐ **E** Sodium valproate

152. A 24-year-old university student has been referred for investigation of constipation. She has had difficulty with her bowels for as long as she can remember. She opens her bowels about once a week and strains at defaecation. She had pain during defaecation, associated with streaks of blood smearing the hard stool, about a month ago. Her General Practitioner has already arranged some blood tests, which are normal. She has no other constitutional symptoms. Which one of the following is true with regards to this patient?

- [ ] **A** Urgent colonoscopy is indicated in view of the rectal bleeding
- [ ] **B** Barium enema is indicated to assess colonic transit
- [ ] **C** Barium enema would be useful to look for megacolon
- [ ] **D** Recto-sigmoid delay in colonic transit suggests a diagnosis of colonic inertia
- [ ] **E** Defaecography is more accurate in the diagnosis of pelvic floor dyssynergia than anorectal manometry

153. A 35-year-old lady is admitted to hospital for a routine cholecystectomy. She is otherwise fit and well, but suffers from a skin condition which is well controlled at present. She makes a good postoperative recovery, but ten days later she notices that her skin condition has developed quite strikingly in her scar site. Which one of the following conditions is she most likely to have?

- [ ] **A** Atopic eczema
- [ ] **B** Dermatitis herpetiformis
- [ ] **C** Discoid lupus erythematosus
- [ ] **D** Dermographism
- [ ] **E** Lichen planus

154. **A 30-year-old man presents with a history of 'funny turns', during which he feels anxious and sweaty. His blood pressure is 160/100 mmHg. Which one of the following investigations would be the best next step in looking for a potentially treatable cause for his hypertension?**

   ☐ **A** 24-hour urine collection for VMA (vanillylmandelic acid)
   ☐ **B** 24-hour urine collection for 5-HIAA
             (5-hydroxyindoleacetic acid)
   ☐ **C** CT scan of the abdomen
   ☐ **D** 24-hour urine collection for catecholamines
   ☐ **E** 24-hour urine collection for urinary free cortisol

155. **A 38-year-old woman saw her doctor complaining of cold, painful fingers. Her fingers turn pale when exposed to cold. She had experienced similar symptoms since she was a teenager. She admits to difficulty in swallowing and progressive shortness of breath for the last six months. Which one of the following statements is true?**

   ☐ **A** Absence of thickened skin anywhere in the body excludes
             the diagnosis of scleroderma
   ☐ **B** Subcutaneous calcification is exclusive to the limited
             cutaneous form (CREST syndrome) and not seen in diffuse
             systemic sclerosis (SSc)
   ☐ **C** In systemic sclerosis the disease course is rarely prolonged
             beyond two years and cure is expected in more than 70%
             of cases
   ☐ **D** Anti-centromere antibodies, when identified, are almost
             diagnostic for limited cutaneous SSc (CREST)
   ☐ **E** Anti-Scl-70 antibodies, when negative, exclude the
             diagnosis of diffuse SSc

156. A 69-year-old man presents with an episode of left-sided pyramidal weakness that resolves within four hours. He has had three similar episodes over the last two years. He takes no medications. On examination he has an irregularly irregular pulse with a rate of 98 bpm. What is the most appropriate management?

- [ ] **A** Aspirin
- [ ] **B** Warfarin
- [ ] **C** Digoxin
- [ ] **D** DC cardioversion
- [ ] **E** Sotalol

157. A 25-year-old man of Asian origin, recently arrived in the UK, is undergoing a routine medical examination. His English is very poor but he does not admit to any previous medical problems. On examination he is pale and has 6 cm of splenomegaly and 3 cm of hepatomegaly. On investigation his haemoglobin is 8.7g/dl, RBC 4.5×10^{12}/l, MCV 65 fl, MCH 23 pg, MCHC 31 g/dl, WCC 5.6×10^9/l, platelets 385×10^9/l. Blood film shows hypochromia, target cells, polychromasia and nucleated red cells. A brilliant cresyl-blue stain reveals red cells with 'golf ball' inclusions. Which one of the following is the diagnosis?

- [ ] **A** β-Thalassaemia major
- [ ] **B** α-Thalassaemia trait
- [ ] **C** Malaria
- [ ] **D** α-Thalassaemia major
- [ ] **E** Haemoglobin H disease

158. A 47-year-old woman presents with bilateral proptosis, chemosis, lid retraction and rapidly worsening visual acuity. What treatment should she be offered?

- [ ] **A** High-dose systemic steroids
- [ ] **B** Carbimazole
- [ ] **C** Radiotherapy
- [ ] **D** Surgical decompression
- [ ] **E** Optic nerve sheath fenestration

159. A 24-year-old Australian backpacker arrives in the UK from travelling throughout sub-Saharan Africa for the previous 12 months. He has a fever, giant urticaria and an eosinophil count of 4.5 × 10⁹/l. How might you best make the diagnosis?

☐ **A** Rectal biopsy
☐ **B** Slit skin smear
☐ **C** Thick blood film
☐ **D** Stool microscopy
☐ **E** Bone marrow examination

160. A 34-year-old woman has been referred by her General Practitioner because of a suspected adverse drug reaction. The patient has a history of treatment-resistant schizophrenia and is prescribed clozapine. Compared to standard antipsychotics, which of one of the following side effects is more common with clozapine?

☐ **A** Acute dystonia
☐ **B** Agranulocytosis
☐ **C** Amenorrhoea
☐ **D** Galactorrhoea
☐ **E** Hyperprolactinaemia

161. A 39-year-old HIV-positive man who smokes presents with cough and haemoptysis. A chest X-ray shows a right upper lobe mass and you proceed to bronchoscopy. Biopsy of the mass shows the presence of carcinoma of the bronchus. Which one of the following is false regarding lung cancer in the context of HIV disease?

☐ **A** Incidence is 3–4 times higher than in the non-HIV population
☐ **B** Adenocarcinoma is the commonest histological subtype
☐ **C** CD4 count of 350 cells/µl is a contraindication to curative resection
☐ **D** Median survival is worse in HIV-positive patients compared to the non-HIV population
☐ **E** HIV patients have smoked more cigarettes than non-HIV patients

162. A 74-year-old man is admitted having collapsed at home. He complains of general malaise and has lost 10 lbs in weight over six months. He is a lifelong smoker and had a single episode of haemoptysis nine days previously. On examination he has a purpuric rash on his legs. Blood pressure is 176/98 mmHg. Dipstick urinalysis demonstrates protein + + + and blood + +. The creatinine is 328 μmol/l, haemoglobin 9.8 g/dl, platelets 204 × 10⁹/l. Which of these statements about his renal failure is correct?

☐ A It is probably due to vasculitis if there is circulating anti-neutrophil cytoplasmic antibody (ANCA) present
☐ B It should be treated with plasma exchange
☐ C It is irreversible
☐ D It is probably secondary to a bronchial neoplasm
☐ E It is due to circulating nephritic factor

163. A 65-year-old lady is seen in a surgical pre-admission clinic prior to her elective urological surgery. She has no past medical problems other than paroxysmal atrial fibrillation (PAF) for which she takes digoxin. The House Officer requests a medical opinion because they are concerned the woman has digoxin toxicity. Which one of the following would support their diagnosis?

☐ A Change in bowel habit
☐ B Persistent atrial fibrillation
☐ C 'Reverse tick' lateral ST-segment depression
☐ D Right axis deviation
☐ E Ventricular ectopics

164. A 21-year-old man presents with an intense frontal headache of sudden onset, with mild photophobia. His temperature is 38 °C and he has meningism. Which one of the following would be more suggestive of a diagnosis of subarachnoid haemorrhage rather than bacterial meningitis?

☐ A History of type I diabetes mellitus
☐ B History of opiate abuse
☐ C Family history of adult polycystic kidney disease
☐ D History of migraine
☐ E Fluctuating level of consciousness

165. A 67-year-old man has a long-standing history of hypertension and diabetes mellitus. Two years ago he suffered a transient ischaemic attack, and aspirin 75 mg daily was commenced. Which one of the following statements best describes its therapeutic pharmacological actions?

☐ A Analgesic effects are due to cyclo-oxygenase inhibition
☐ B Increased renal urate reabsorption
☐ C Inhibition of thromboxane A_2 synthesis by platelets
☐ D Recovery of platelet function takes about 24–48 hours
☐ E Reduced activation of factor V

166. A CT scan of the brain of a 35-year-old Asian woman shows at least seven ring-enhancing lesions, each about 1.5 cm in diameter and with surrounding oedema. She gives a five-day history of high fevers, rigors, myalgia, malaise and a headache, and has just had a fit. What is the most likely diagnosis?

☐ A Multiple cerebral tuberculomas
☐ B Cerebral toxoplasmosis related to HIV
☐ C Multiple staphylococcal abscesses
☐ D Cerebral cysticercosis
☐ E Herpes simplex virus (HSV) encephalitis

167. A 53-year-old man is currently receiving treatment as an inpatient at the local hospice. He has noticed a scaly thickening of the skin on his palms and soles in the past few months. On examination, there is an even, very thick, yellow hyperkeratosis affecting the soles and palms with a sharp cut-off at the wrist. His nails are also slightly thickened but there is no evidence of dystrophy. What is the most likely underlying diagnosis?

☐ A Acute myeloid leukaemia
☐ B Bronchial carcinoma
☐ C Oesophageal carcinoma
☐ D Lymphoma
☐ E Glucagonoma

168. A 23-year-old medical student develops a viral upper respiratory tract infection and notices that his urine becomes very dark. On entry to medical school urinalysis had been unremarkable. His GP repeats the urinalysis, demonstrating blood +++ but no protein. Blood pressure is 124/74 mmHg. Examination is unremarkable. All routine investigations are normal. What is the most likely diagnosis?

- [ ] **A** Henoch-Schönlein syndrome
- [ ] **B** Mesangial IgA disease
- [ ] **C** Acute tubular necrosis
- [ ] **D** Rhabdomyolysis
- [ ] **E** Membranous glomerulonephropathy

169. A 64-year-old man had a mitral valve replacement three years ago. He attends the Anticoagulant Clinic two days after his daughter's wedding where he consumed a considerable quantity of alcohol. He has a history of previous excess alcohol intake. His INR is found to be 8.5. He has a few bruises on his legs and on testing he has 3+ of microscopic haematuria. Which one of the following is the most appropriate immediate management of his condition?

- [ ] **A** Give 0.5 mg vitamin K intravenously
- [ ] **B** Give 10 mg vitamin K intravenously
- [ ] **C** Give 2 units of fresh frozen plasma
- [ ] **D** Observe the patient only
- [ ] **E** Give 2 units of cryoprecipitate

170. An 18-year-old girl is referred for the investigations of raised liver enzymes. She had type 1 diabetes diagnosed in 1993. For the first six years glycaemic control was good with Hb A$_{1c}$ just above 6%. She developed ketoacidosis in June 2000, when she was noted to have macrocytosis and abnormal liver tests. Since then she has had a further two episodes of ketoacidosis. Her attendance at the clinic had become inconsistent and her Hb A$_{1c}$ was 14.7% and 16.3% at her last two visits. She had been taking quite high doses of insulin and insists that she never misses her insulin. There has been a noticeable change in her weight, which fluctuated between 58 kg and 70 kg. She denies alcohol intake. On examination there were no stigmata of chronic liver disease. Systemic examination was normal. Investigations: haemoglobin 14.9 g/dl, WCC 6.5 × 10^9 /l, platelets 410 × 10^9/l, MCV 99.3 fl.

Date	Nov/01	Jan/02	May/02	Normal
Albumin	45	43	44	37–49 g/l
Bilirubin	9	12	11	<22 μmol/l
ALP	284	280	438	20–120 U/l
ALT	29	160	314	<35 U/l
GGT	277	479	1316	<4–35 U/l

Immunoglobulins normal; autoantibody profile negative; serology for hepatitis B and C negative; serum copper on two occasions 28 μmol/l; caeruloplasmin on two occasions 120 mg/l. Ultrasound abdomen: liver is enlarged; spleen, both kidneys and pancreas appear normal. Which one of the following is true when the diagnosis of Wilson's disease is suspected?

☐ A Estimation of hepatic copper concentration is the definitive test to establish the diagnosis of Wilson's disease

☐ B Genotyping for the *ATP7B* gene is the most sensitive investigation

☐ C Absence of Kayser-Fleischer rings on slit–lamp examination would exclude the diagnosis of Wilson's disease in patients with hepatic manifestations

☐ D Low serum caeruloplasmin is more sensitive in patients who present with acute hepatic failure

☐ E Urinary copper estimation is more useful in the diagnosis than for monitoring treatment

171. A 26-year-old woman has been admitted, having collapsed on a street. The history from the patient indicates a possible eating disorder as a cause of her presentation. Which one of the following is least important for the diagnosis of bulimia nervosa?

- [ ] **A** Repeated attempts to reduce the fattening effects of food
- [ ] **B** Body image distortion
- [ ] **C** Craving for food
- [ ] **D** Episodes of overeating
- [ ] **E** Fear of fatness

172. A 45-year-old man presents with dyspnoea when going swimming. On further questioning you find out that it is worse when he is walking into the water but improves once he starts swimming. Which one of the following investigations is likely to give you the correct diagnosis?

- [ ] **A** Transoesophageal echocardiogram
- [ ] **B** Ventilation–perfusion ($\dot{V}/\dot{Q}$) scanning
- [ ] **C** Transdiaphragmatic pressure measurement
- [ ] **D** High-resolution computed tomography (CT)
- [ ] **E** Right heart catheterisation

173. A 39-year-old male decorator complains of hand pain. Radiographs of both hands are notable for degenerative changes in the second and third metacarpophalangeal joints. Which one of the following is the most helpful diagnostic test?

- [ ] **A** Erythrocyte sedimentation rate (ESR)
- [ ] **B** Uric acid levels
- [ ] **C** Ferritin level
- [ ] **D** Antinuclear antibody
- [ ] **E** Rheumatoid factor

174. A 38-year-old woman presents with a tremor of her left hand that is particularly noticeable when holding objects and when she is stressed at work. Her mother had a similar tremor of both hands. What is the most appropriate treatment for her condition?

☐ **A** Levodopa
☐ **B** Selegiline
☐ **C** Propranolol
☐ **D** Pizotifen
☐ **E** Botulinum toxin

175. A 40-year-old HIV-positive man initially presented 18 months ago with a CD4 count of 25 cells/µl and viral load of 150,000 copies/ml. He was started on cotrimoxazole, zidovudine, lamivudine and efavirenz and has responded well. His CD4 count six months ago had risen to 250 cells/µl and is now 275 cells/µl. His viral load has been undetectable for the past year. Which one of the following may he now do safely?

☐ **A** Discontinue the cotrimoxazole
☐ **B** Rationalise his antiretroviral therapy by discontinuing the efavirenz
☐ **C** Have unprotected intercourse without fear of infecting his partner
☐ **D** Return to work as a general surgeon
☐ **E** Receive BCG vaccination

176. An 80-year-old lady is admitted from the Accident and Emergency Department with falls. Cardiac monitoring during her admission is performed and shows runs of fast atrial fibrillation as well as pauses which are associated with dizzy spells. A diagnosis of sick sinus syndrome is made and a dual chamber pacemaker is implanted. Which one of the following is true of the sinoatrial node?

☐ **A** Action potentials are triggered by the opening of sodium channels
☐ **B** Automaticity is mediated by calcium channels
☐ **C** Vagotomy results in a loss of automaticity
☐ **D** Sodium efflux restores the resting potential
☐ **E** Potassium influx is triggers the action potential

177. Which one of the following statements regarding verapamil is correct?

- [ ] **A** It is a dihydropyridine-type calcium-channel blocker
- [ ] **B** It enhances slow Ca^{2+} entry to myocardial cells
- [ ] **C** It can be administered orally or intravenously
- [ ] **D** It is safe in patients with sinoatrial disease
- [ ] **E** It has oral bioavailability of around 75%

178. Children with otitis media are randomised to receive either a long or a short course of antibiotics. The numbers who have recurrent attacks within the following 12 months are compared. Which one of the following is the most appropriate statistical test to make this comparison:

- [ ] **A** Analysis of variance
- [ ] **B** Chi-square test
- [ ] **C** Student's *t*-test
- [ ] **D** Mann-Whitney *U* test
- [ ] **E** Regression analysis

179. A 21-year-old lady presents with malaise, fever and arthralgia. She also complains of painful hot lumps on her legs. She is not on any medication. On examination there are tender, erythematous nodules present on both anterior shins. Skin biopsy demonstrates inflammation in the subcutaneous fat. What is the most important investigation to perform?

- [ ] **A** Chest X-ray
- [ ] **B** Serum glucose
- [ ] **C** Urinalysis
- [ ] **D** Arterial blood gases
- [ ] **E** ESR

180. A 35-year-old lady presents with thyrotoxicosis. Which one of the following physical signs best supports a diagnosis of Graves' disease?

☐ **A** Ophthalmoplegia
☐ **B** Lid retraction
☐ **C** Tremor
☐ **D** Atrial fibrillation
☐ **E** Symmetrical goitre

181. A ten-year-old Pakistani boy is referred for investigation of anaemia. He is well but is smaller than his younger siblings. On examination he is pale and has a number of *café-au-lait* spots on his back. On laboratory investigation his haemoglobin is 8.2 g/dl, WCC 2.4 × 10⁹/l with a normal differential, and platelets 22 × 10⁹/l. What is the most likely diagnosis?

☐ **A** Idiopathic aplastic anaemia
☐ **B** Acute lymphoblastic leukaemia
☐ **C** Diamond-Blackfan syndrome
☐ **D** Fanconi's anaemia
☐ **E** Congenital dyserythropoietic anaemia

182. A 36-year-old black woman presents with gradual onset of 'floaters' and mildly reduced visual acuity in both eyes (6/12 right and left). What is the most likely diagnosis?

☐ **A** Tuberculosis
☐ **B** Ulcerative colitis
☐ **C** Behçet's disease
☐ **D** Ankylosing spondylitis
☐ **E** Sarcoidosis

183. A 28-year-old female marathon runner is found to have dipstick haematuria at a routine medical. No protein is detected. Pulse is 54 bpm, blood pressure is 110/64 mmHg. Examination is unremarkable. All investigations are normal. Renal biopsy demonstrates mild mesangial hypercellularity with mesangial IgA deposition on immunostaining. Which of these statements about this renal disease is correct?

- [ ] A It is the commonest primary glomerulonephritis leading to renal failure
- [ ] B It has a 50% chance of progressing to end-stage renal failure over 20 years
- [ ] C It is associated with hepatitis B infection
- [ ] D More commonly it presents with nephrotic syndrome
- [ ] E It can be associated with crescentic glomerulonephritis

184. A 50-year-old woman presented with vomiting coffee-ground fluid a few times on the day of admission. After initial investigations and fluid resuscitation she underwent an upper gastrointestinal endoscopy which showed an ulcer, 1 cm in diameter, in the duodenal cap. The rapid urease test was positive. Which one of the following is the most appropriate next step in her management?

- [ ] A Treatment with a combination of a proton pump inhibitor, amoxicillin and clarithromycin
- [ ] B Lifelong maintenance treatment with proton pump inhibitors to prevent recurrence
- [ ] C Upper gastrointestinal endoscopy to be repeated in six weeks' time to confirm healing
- [ ] D Serology for IgG antibody to *Helicobacter pylori* in six weeks' time to confirm *H. pylori* eradication
- [ ] E Urease breath test to confirm *H. pylori* eradication before discontinuation of proton pump inhibitors

185. A 54-year-old woman at a follow-up appointment insists that you repeat an endoscopy, despite recent negative findings on investigation. She states her husband is trying to secretly poison her and complains of abdominal pain. You perform a mental state examination as she might benefit from an antipsychotic. Which one of the following lends least weight to a diagnosis of a delusional disorder (paranoid psychosis)?

☐ **A** An unshakeable belief that her husband is trying to poison her
☐ **B** Feeling a burning sensation over her abdomen
☐ **C** Hearing third person hallucinations discussing her children
☐ **D** The belief has been present for three months
☐ **E** The belief is untrue

186. A 65-year-old man with chronic obstructive pulmonary disease (COPD) is referred for pulmonary rehabilitation. He is receiving maximal medical therapy including long-term oxygen therapy. Which one of the following statements concerning pulmonary rehabilitation in COPD are false?

☐ **A** Benefits are independent of age
☐ **B** Benefits are dependent on FEV_1
☐ **C** Benefits are independent of oxygen dependence
☐ **D** Benefits are independent of associated disease
☐ **E** Benefits include decreased number of hospitalisations

187. A 42-year-old guitarist presents with a three-month history of pain and weakness in the right thumb of gradual onset. He describes altered sensation in the thumb and difficulty opening bottles and jars. There are no problems in the other limbs and no history of trauma. On examination there is weakness of right forearm pronation and flexion of the distal phalanges of thumb and right index finger; sensation is normal. Which structure is most likely to be damaged?

☐ **A** Anterior interosseous nerve
☐ **B** Median nerve
☐ **C** Ulnar nerve
☐ **D** Lower cord of the brachial plexus
☐ **E** C4 nerve root

188. A 35-year-old Caucasian teacher presents with back pain. He states that his lower back has been increasingly painful over the past four months. The symptoms are worse in the morning and after naps. He gave up his job as he used to have to get up very early in the morning to allow the stiffness to settle before he set off to school. Which one of the following results will virtually exclude the diagnosis of ankylosing spondylitis?

- [ ] **A** Low antinuclear antibody (ANA) titre
- [ ] **B** Normal chest X-rays
- [ ] **C** Absent HLA-B27 gene
- [ ] **D** Normal DEXA scan
- [ ] **E** Negative plain sacroiliac radiographs

189. A 50-year-old woman with a primary dilated cardiomyopathy presents to Casualty with severe shortness of breath. She has had several similar episodes in the past, requiring intravenous diuretics. She takes regular ramipril, spironolactone, bisoprolol, furosemide (frusemide) and warfarin. On examination her pulse is 110 bpm, thready in character, her blood pressure is 80/30 mmHg, her JVP is raised and she has crepitations to the mid-zones.
She is commenced on inotropic support. Concerning positive inotropes:

- [ ] **A** Dobutamine exerts its action through α-adrenergic receptors
- [ ] **B** Dopamine acts mainly through nicotinic receptors
- [ ] **C** Noradrenaline (norepinephrine) has greater potency on α receptors than on β receptors
- [ ] **D** Milrinone acts selectively on β receptors
- [ ] **E** Adrenaline (epinephrine) is less selective than noradrenaline

190. Which one of the following is a recognised pharmacological effect of nifedipine?

- [ ] **A** Increased cardiac afterload
- [ ] **B** Increased peripheral capillary pressure
- [ ] **C** Increased vascular sensitivity to nitrates
- [ ] **D** Reduced cardiac output
- [ ] **E** Reduced cardiovascular sympathetic activity

191. A 72-year-old woman with congestive cardiac failure is treated with regular bumetanide to improve her clinical symptoms. Which one of the following is NOT a recognised adverse effect of bumetanide treatment?

- ☐ **A** Hypertriglyceridaemia
- ☐ **B** Hyperuricaemia
- ☐ **C** Hypomagnesaemia
- ☐ **D** Metabolic alkalosis
- ☐ **E** Raised serum urea concentration

192. A 33-year-old man presents with a skin eruption affecting his face, scalp and chest. It has been deteriorating over the past few months. He is HIV-positive and is currently on zidovudine. On examination, he has a red, scaly eruption on his scalp, ears, nasolabial folds, and eyebrows. There are also dry, scaly areas in the presternal and interscapular areas with extensive follicular papules. What is the most likely diagnosis?

- ☐ **A** Atopic eczema
- ☐ **B** Kaposi's sarcoma
- ☐ **C** Rosacea
- ☐ **D** Seborrhoeic eczema
- ☐ **E** Herpes zoster

193. A security guard in a supermarket is bitten during a scuffle by an intravenous drug user as he is attempting to apprehend him. The bite draws blood. The shoplifter appears to be bleeding from his mouth as he runs out of the store. Which of the following would be LEAST useful to offer to the security guard when he presents at the Accident and Emergency Department?

- ☐ **A** Co-amoxiclav
- ☐ **B** HIV post-exposure prophylaxis (HAART)
- ☐ **C** Hepatitis B post-exposure prophylaxis (vaccine +/–immunoglobulin)
- ☐ **D** Hepatitis C post-exposure prophylaxis (interferon and ribavirin)
- ☐ **E** Tetanus post-exposure prophylaxis (vaccine+/–immunoglobulin)

194. A 60-year-old man has had type 2 diabetes for five years. He had been diet-controlled until six months ago, when his GP started metformin. He now sees his GP complaining of diarrhoea. Which one of the following is the most likely cause of his diarrhoea?

☐ **A** Diabetic autonomic neuropathy
☐ **B** Coeliac disease
☐ **C** Metformin therapy
☐ **D** Irritable bowel syndrome
☐ **E** Colon cancer

195. A 23-year-old woman has recently suffered a first trimester abortion. She is still feeling tired and unwell and attends her General Practitioner. In her history she has had two normal deliveries and 2 first trimester abortions over a six-year period. She is pale but there is nothing to find on examination. The GP orders some investigations, the results of which are as follows: haemoglobin 8.8 g/dl, MCV 69 fl, MCH 25 pg, MCHC 28 g/dl, WCC 9.5 × 10⁹/l, platelets 632 × 10⁹/l, normal urea and electrolytes and liver function tests, serum iron 8 μmol/l (normal range 14–29 μmol/l), TIBC 80 μmol/l (normal range 45–72 μmol/l), ferritin 8 μg/l (normal range 15–200 μg/l). Her coagulation screen is entirely normal. Why is her platelet count raised?

☐ **A** Primary thrombocythaemia
☐ **B** Reactive thrombocytosis
☐ **C** Chronic myeloid leukaemia
☐ **D** Myelofibrosis
☐ **E** Polycythaemia rubra vera

196. A 55-year-old woman has presented to the Accident and Emergency Department with palpitations, tachycardia and chest discomfort. An ECG reveals no evidence of ischaemia. On further questioning the patient admits to a history of paroxysmal attacks of palpitations accompanied by tremor, dyspnoea and nausea. You wish to exclude panic disorder as a possible cause for her symptoms. Which one of the following psychological symptoms would most support this diagnosis?

- [ ] **A** Constant fear that something terrible will happen
- [ ] **B** Fear of crowded places
- [ ] **C** Fear that she has a serious underlying physical illness
- [ ] **D** Fear that she will lose control of herself during an attack
- [ ] **E** Inability to be reassured that there is no organic illness present

197. A 64-year-old woman with end-stage renal failure treated by haemodialysis develops shingles, which is treated with oral aciclovir 400 mg × 5 daily and codeine phosphate analgesia. All other medications are continued unchanged. Three days later she is found unrousable with a Glasgow Coma Scale score of 4, pulse 76 bpm, blood pressure 134/76 mmHg, temperature 37.4 °C. Pupils are small but reactive to light and the cranial nerves are intact. Neurological examination demonstrates no focal neurology. Examination is otherwise unremarkable. Urgent magnetic resonance imaging (MRI) of the head demonstrates no acute abnormality. What is the most likely cause of this patient's confusional state?

- [ ] **A** Dialysis dysequilibrium syndrome
- [ ] **B** Aciclovir toxicity
- [ ] **C** Opiate toxicity
- [ ] **D** Cerebrovascular accident
- [ ] **E** Encephalitis

198. A 44-year-old man with a history of alcohol and intravenous drug abuse presents with abdominal distension and is found to have ascites. Diagnostic paracentesis is performed and ascitic fluid is analysed. The peritoneal fluid analysis shows: albumin 10 g/l (serum albumin 26 g/l), glucose 3 mmol/l (serum glucose 6.5 mmol/l), LDH 250 U/l (serum LDH 200 U/l), neutrophil count > 500 cells/mm³, creamy appearance. What is the most likely diagnosis?

- ☐ **A** Cirrhosis with portal hypertension
- ☐ **B** Spontaneous bacterial peritonitis
- ☐ **C** Acute pancreatitis
- ☐ **D** Tuberculous peritonitis
- ☐ **E** Chylous ascites

199. A 37-year-old woman presents with a two-week history of gradually worsening vision in the left eye, accompanied by discomfort on eye movements. Visual acuity is 6/60 on the left with impaired colour vision on Ishihara testing. There is a left afferent pupillary defect and a central scotoma on Goldman perimetry. Eye movements are full but accompanied by mild discomfort. What is the most likely diagnosis?

- ☐ **A** Optic nerve glioma
- ☐ **B** Cavernous sinus thrombosis
- ☐ **C** Graves' disease
- ☐ **D** Pituitary adenoma
- ☐ **E** Optic neuritis

200. A 39-year-old man with asthma takes a number of medications, including salmeterol and salbutamol. Salmeterol demonstrates a number of differences from salbutamol. Which one of the following statements about salmeterol compared to salbutamol is false?

- ☐ **A** Salmeterol has lower lipophilicity
- ☐ **B** Salmeterol has greater bronchial tissue penetration
- ☐ **C** Salmeterol has greater resistance to its own metabolism
- ☐ **D** Salmeterol has slower clearance from the airways
- ☐ **E** Salmeterol binds to β_2-adrenoceptors

201. A 63-year-old man is referred to hospital because of cough, wheezing, dyspnoea, and fever. He has a 16-year history of severe asthma. Lower respiratory tract infection with asthma exacerbation is diagnosed. His white blood cell (WBC) count is $32 \times 10^9/l$ (normal range $4-11 \times 10^9/l$) with 55% eosinophils (normal range 0–7%). Chest radiography revealed bilateral alveolar infiltrates. While in hospital he developed multiple discrete ecchymotic macules scattered on his arms, lower torso, and lower extremities. One week later he developed parasthesiae in the distal arms and legs which progressed to a left wrist drop and bilateral foot drop. Which one of the following is the most likely cause of this patient's eosinophilia and pulmonary infiltrates?

☐ **A** Chronic eosinophilic pneumonia
☐ **B** Allergic bronchopulmonary aspergillosis
☐ **C** Parasitic infection
☐ **D** Vasculitis
☐ **E** Idiopathic hypereosinophilic syndrome (IHS)

202. A 42-year-old male smoker presents with chest pain on exertion. His GP suspects angina and refers him for exercise testing which is positive for ST changes and symptoms after 5 h 24 min. A cardiac catheter is arranged and stenoses are seen in the left anterior descending, circumflex and right coronary arteries. Which one of the following is true of the normal coronary circulation?

☐ **A** The left anterior descending and left circumflex arteries arise from the coronary sinus
☐ **B** The right coronary artery usually gives rise to the posterior descending artery
☐ **C** The septum is supplied by branches of the left circumflex artery
☐ **D** The sinoatrial node is usually supplied by branches of the left anterior descending artery
☐ **E** The intermediate artery is an occasional feature arising above the non-coronary cusp of the aortic valve

203. A 70-year-old man has a long history of hypertension and has been taking aspirin 75 mg daily, and atenolol 50 mg daily for ten years with no reported side effects. He is found to have evidence of congestive cardiac failure. Which one of the following drugs should be added to his current drug regimen to reduce the risk of future cardiovascular disease (myocardial infarction and stroke)?

- [ ] **A** Digoxin
- [ ] **B** Doxazosin
- [ ] **C** Furosemide (frusemide)
- [ ] **D** Isosorbide dinitrate
- [ ] **E** Lisinopril

204. A 40-year-old man is found the have a high cholesterol. Which one of the following features best supports a diagnosis of familial hypercholesterolaemia?

- [ ] **A** His total cholesterol is 8 mmol/l
- [ ] **B** He has impaired glucose tolerance
- [ ] **C** His father died of a myocardial infarction at the age of 65
- [ ] **D** He has tendon xanthomata
- [ ] **E** He has primary hypothyroidism

205. A 35-year-old man has been ventilated in the Intensive Care Unit for nine weeks following a road traffic accident in which he sustained extensive chest and abdominal injuries. His recovery has been slow and complicated by ongoing sepsis. He is noted over the course of the last week to be becoming progressively anaemic despite there being no source of blood loss. His haemoglobin is 5.4 g/dl, MCV 110 fl, WCC 2.5 × 10⁹/l, platelets 120 × 10⁹/l. He has mild stable renal and hepatic impairment. What is the most likely cause of his anaemia?

- [ ] **A** Acute myeloid leukaemia
- [ ] **B** Occult blood loss
- [ ] **C** Acute folic acid deficiency
- [ ] **D** Aplastic anaemia
- [ ] **E** Systemic lupus erythematosus

206. A 14-year-old boy has returned from a rural camping holiday in Wales with his classmates. He has become very unwell, with a fever. He is jaundiced, has conjunctival suffusion and hepatosplenomegaly and has developed acute renal failure. What is the most likely diagnosis?

☐ **A** Q fever
☐ **B** Lyme disease
☐ **C** Haemolytic-uraemic syndrome (HUS)
☐ **D** Brucellosis
☐ **E** Leptospirosis

207. A 42-year-old patient with end-stage renal failure has been treated with haemodialysis for 12 years. Routine screening demonstrates a haemoglobin of 9.2 g/dl, WCC 4.3 × 10^9/l, platelet count of 230 × 10^9/l and MCV 88 fl. Ferritin is 190 μg/l with hypochromic red blood cells of 1.2%. Folate and vitamin B$_{12}$ levels are normal. He takes perindopril 8 mg once daily, atenolol 50 mg once daily, alphacalcidol 250 ng × 3 each week, aluminium hydroxide 2 tabs tds and erythropoietin beta 4000 units × 3 each week. What is the most likely cause of his anaemia?

☐ **A** Haemolysis in the dialysis circuit
☐ **B** Iron deficiency
☐ **C** Erythropoietin deficiency
☐ **D** Aluminium toxicity
☐ **E** Pure red cell aplasia (PRCA)

208. A 58-year-old woman presents with intermittent indigestion of four months' duration. She has no nausea. Her appetite remains good and she has not lost weight. Her past medical history includes stable angina and hypertension for which she is taking atenolol and aspirin. She was started on ibuprofen for osteoarthritis six months ago. Which one of the following is true regarding the mechanism of action of non-steroidal anti-inflammatory drugs (NSAIDs)?

   ☐ A Gastrointestinal injury from aspirin is entirely due to inhibition of prostaglandin synthesis
   ☐ B Enteric coating of NSAIDs prevents the occurrence of ulcers in chronic NSAID users
   ☐ C The Cyclo-oxygenase 1 (COX-1) enzyme is produced in response to inflammation
   ☐ D The COX-1 enzyme is involved in mucosal protection
   ☐ E COX-2-specific NSAIDs inhibit platelet aggregation

209. A 44-year-old woman is admitted from the clinic. You think that she has an acute eosinophilic pneumonia, as she has had a similar episode previously. Which one of the following features would you be least likely to find in acute eosinophilic pneumonia?

   ☐ A Multilobar consolidation on chest X-ray
   ☐ B Normal blood eosinophil count
   ☐ C Gradual response to high-dose corticosteroids
   ☐ D Bronchoalveolar lavage eosinophil count > 25%
   ☐ E Restrictive ventilatory defect

210. A 36-year-old man with asthma since childhood has been treated with multiple courses of prednisolone over the years, with durations ranging from a week to many months at a time. About a year ago, his inhaled steroid dose was increased, and subsequently he has not required systemic glucocorticoids. Which one of the following statements is most correct?

- [ ] **A** Treatment with bisphosphonate should be commenced without delay
- [ ] **B** Being male, the risk for osteoporosis is negligible
- [ ] **C** In the absence of prednisolone for a year, he is no longer at risk for osteoporosis
- [ ] **D** Inhaled steroids alone do not affect the risk of osteoporosis
- [ ] **E** He may have osteoporosis and dual energy X-ray absorptiometry (DEXA) should be arranged

211. An 82-year-old woman presents to the orthopaedic surgeons with a right fractured neck of femur. She admits to a long history of dizzy spells and falls. A cardiology opinion is requested and trifascicular block noted on her resting ECG. No reversible cause is found and a dual chamber pacemaker is implanted. Which one of the following ECGs would most support a diagnosis of trifascicular block?

- [ ] **A** Left bundle branch block and left axis deviation
- [ ] **B** First-degree atrioventricular block and left bundle branch block
- [ ] **C** Right bundle branch block and left axis deviation
- [ ] **D** First-degree atrioventricular block and right bundle branch block
- [ ] **E** Left anterior hemiblock

212. A 58-year-old woman is diagnosed with angina, and several new treatments have been commenced. Which one of the following drugs has NOT been proved to reduce future cardiovascular morbidity or mortality?

- [ ] **A** Aspirin
- [ ] **B** Atenolol
- [ ] **C** Nifedipine
- [ ] **D** Ramipril
- [ ] **E** Simvastatin

213. A 54-year-old man attends with a suspicious lesion on his forearm. He has a lifelong history of atopic eczema and has been treated in the past with frequent courses of PUVA therapy. Which one of the following lesions is he most at risk of having developed?

☐ A Squamous cell carcinoma
☐ B Seborrhoeic keratosis
☐ C Superficial spreading malignant melanoma
☐ D Pyoderma gangrenosum
☐ E Pyogenic granuloma

214. A dentist refers a 43-year-old man to the Endocrine Clinic suspecting possible acromegaly. Which one of the following is the 'gold standard' diagnostic test for this condition?

☐ A A 24-hour urine collection for growth hormone
☐ B Oral glucose tolerance test with measurement of growth hormone concentrations
☐ C Serum insulin-like growth factor-1 (IGF-1) concentration
☐ D 9 am growth hormone concentration
☐ E Serum IGF-binding protein 3 (IGF-BP3) concentration

215. A three-day-old baby boy has a raised white cell count about which you are consulted. The baby was born prematurely at 30 weeks and has been in Paediatric Intensive Care with respiratory distress and sepsis since birth. He continues to require ventilatory support, intravenous antibiotics, inotropes and intensive support. His full blood count is as follows: haemoglobin 11.5 g/dl, WCC 85 × 10⁹/l, blasts 3%, promyelocytes 5%, myelocytes 34%, metamyelocytes 15%, neutrophils 43%, and platelets 124 × 10⁹/l. Blood film shows 10 nucleated RBCs per 100 WBCs. Which one of the following is the most likely cause of the raised white cell count?

☐ A Acute myeloid leukaemia
☐ B Chronic myeloid leukaemia
☐ C β-Thalassaemia major
☐ D Leukaemoid reaction
☐ E Acute lymphoblastic leukaemia

216. A 57-year-old woman with rheumatoid arthritis is commenced on hydroxychloroquine. Which statement is correct regarding this treatment?

- ☐ **A** There is a substantial risk of toxicity
- ☐ **B** Fundoscopic changes can be used to predict progression to visual loss
- ☐ **C** Colour vision should be monitored
- ☐ **D** Toxicity is idiosyncratic and not dose-related
- ☐ **E** Changes are reversible on cessation of the hydroxychloroquine

217. A 28-year-old man has presented to the Accident and Emergency Department after being injured in a fight. You find it hard to interrupt his speech and he appears irritable. Which one of the following would most suggest that this gentleman is suffering from a hypomanic episode?

- ☐ **A** Hearing God's voice in the form of a hallucination
- ☐ **B** Persistent elevation of mood
- ☐ **C** Persistent reduction of energy levels
- ☐ **D** Repeated episodes of aggression
- ☐ **E** Unshakeable belief that he is the reincarnation of Bruce Lee

218. A 64-year-old man presents with a two-day history of sudden-onset frontal headache and vertigo, and a one-day history of intermittent horizontal diplopia. Six hours before admission he collapsed at home and was admitted. On examination he is mildly febrile (37.9 °C), and has a Glasgow Coma Scale score of 7. Pupils are 4 mm and sluggishly reactive, with a convergent strabismus. Fundoscopy is normal and there is no neck stiffness. He is moving all four limbs, with brisk reflexes and upgoing plantars. Urgent CT and limited MRI (T1 and T2 sequences) studies are normal. What is the most important next step in this man's management?

- ☐ **A** Immediate treatment with intravenous methylprednisolone
- ☐ **B** Urgent magnetic resonance angiogram
- ☐ **C** Urgent lumbar puncture
- ☐ **D** Immediate treatment with intravenous heparin
- ☐ **E** Immediate treatment with intravenous nimodipine

219. A 25-year-old man develops acute encephalitis six months after returning to the UK from India. Magnetic resonance imaging of the brain is unremarkable. PCR of cerebrospinal fluid is negative for herpes simplex virus, varicella zoster virus and enteroviruses. A viral aetiology is considered probable. What is the most likely diagnosis?

- [ ] **A** Rabies
- [ ] **B** Japanese encephalitis
- [ ] **C** West Nile virus
- [ ] **D** Human T-lymphotropic virus 1 (HTLV-1)
- [ ] **E** Tick-borne encephalitis

220. A 36-year-old man consults his GP with symptoms suggestive of a viral upper respiratory tract infection and is found to have a blood pressure of 186/98 mmHg. Dipstick urinalysis reveals blood +++ and protein ++. Haemoglobin is 10.8 g/dl, sodium 136 mmol/l, potassium 3.8 mmol/l, urea 14.8 mmol/l and creatinine 240 µmol/l. Albumin is 40 g/dl, with a 24-hour urinary protein excretion of 0.7 g. Ultrasound scan demonstrates both kidneys to be 8.4 cm, with a bright appearance of the cortex and no pelvicalyceal dilatation. Which one of the following statements is true?

- [ ] **A** The most likely diagnosis is post-infectious glomerulonephritis
- [ ] **B** The ultrasound appearances are typical of acute renal failure
- [ ] **C** Demonstration of C3 nephritic factor would suggest a diagnosis of mesangiocapillary glomerulonephritis
- [ ] **D** Demonstration of spikes on renal biopsy would suggest a diagnosis of membranous glomerulonephropathy
- [ ] **E** There is a 50% chance of his children inheriting this renal disease

221. A 46-year-old man with a diagnosis of hepatitis C cirrhosis has been referred for consideration of liver transplantation. Which one of the following is the best indicator of long-term prognosis in patients with cirrhosis?

☐ **A** Degree of dependent oedema
☐ **B** Mean corpuscular volume (MCV)
☐ **C** Prothrombin time
☐ **D** Alanine transaminase
☐ **E** Alkaline phosphatase

222. You decide to give inhaled corticosteroids to a 62-year-old woman with chronic obstructive pulmonary disease (COPD). She is a little reluctant, as a friend of hers from the Bridge Club developed oral candidiasis and a hoarse voice when she took inhaled corticosteroids. You explain to her that fluticasone propionate (FP) can be used at a lower dose while maintaining the beneficial effects. Which one of the following statements regarding the use of inhaled fluticasone (compared to placebo) in COPD is false?

☐ **A** Exacerbation rates are decreased by 25%
☐ **B** Rate of decline in quality of life is decreased
☐ **C** There is no relationship between acute and chronic steroid responses
☐ **D** Post-bronchodilator FEV_1 is significantly increased
☐ **E** Rate of decline of post-bronchodilator FEV_1 is significantly decreased

223. A 78-year-old lady presents with difficulty chewing food, especially meat, for the last two months. She also admits to feeling pressure and pain in the jaw, even when talking. She has intermittent headache and has lost one stone in weight. The ESR was at 105 mm/hr. Which one of the following tests is the most appropriate?

☐ **A** Electrocardiogram (ECG)
☐ **B** Plain X-ray of the mandible
☐ **C** Temporal artery biopsy
☐ **D** Parotid sialogram
☐ **E** CT scan of the brain

224. A 58-year-old male gardener with known mitral valve prolapse presents to his GP having failed to recover from a chest infection that he had three weeks ago. It initially responded to amoxicillin but, although his cough subsided, the malaise returned after stopping the amoxicillin. On examination, his temperature is 37.4 °C, pulse 82 bpm, blood pressure 140/80 mmHg, he has three splinter haemorrhages, and his GP suspects his murmur is louder than before. His dipstick urinalysis shows blood++. Infective endocarditis is suspected and he is admitted that evening to the local hospital. What is the most important aspect of his initial management?

☐ A Immediate referral to the nearest cardiology tertiary centre for transoesophageal echocardiography

☐ B Commence ampicillin and gentamicin after taking six sets of blood cultures

☐ C Multiple blood cultures and discharge home with a temperature chart and thermometer, to be called with the result

☐ D Multiple blood cultures and observation in hospital pending the result

☐ E Discharge home on oral amoxicillin with a thermometer and temperature chart

225. A 60-year-old man is diagnosed with sustained hypertension. Which one of the following drug combinations is potentially hazardous and should be avoided?

☐ A Bendroflumethazide (bendrofluazide) and doxazosin
☐ B Bisoprolol and lisinopril
☐ C Diltiazem and atenolol
☐ D Nifedipine and enalapril
☐ E Verapamil and enalapril

226. A 26-year-old lady presents with a six-month history of red lesions appearing on her cheeks and ears. She has recently noticed an area developing on her scalp, and is concerned because her scalp is now bald in this area. She has noticed that the lesions get worse in sunshine. On examination, there are well-demarcated erythematous plaques which are slightly scaly, with some follicular plugging. There is also some scarring of the scalp. Which one of the following diagnoses is most likely?

☐ **A** Gorlin's syndrome
☐ **B** Dermatomyositis
☐ **C** Morphoea
☐ **D** Polymorphic light eruption
☐ **E** Discoid lupus erythematosus

227. A 50-year-old man presents with erectile dysfunction. He is found to have a prolactin-secreting pituitary macroadenoma. Formal assessment of his visual fields reveals bi-temporal upper quadrantanopia. Which one of the following is the preferred first-line treatment?

☐ **A** Trans-sphenoidal resection of the pituitary adenoma
☐ **B** Pituitary radiotherapy
☐ **C** Testosterone
☐ **D** Sildenafil (Viagra®)
☐ **E** A dopamine agonist (e.g. bromocriptine or cabergoline)

228. A 70-year-old woman presents with a history of weight loss and generalised lymphadenopathy. A cervical lymph node biopsy is non-diagnostic. Her haemoglobin is 12.4 g/dl, WCC 12.6 × 10⁹/l, platelets 157 × 10⁹/l, neutrophils 4.5 × 10⁹/l, lymphocytes 6.0 ×10⁹/l and monocytes 1.1 × 10⁹/l. A bone marrow examination is carried out. Which one of the following tests on the bone marrow may show that the lymphocytosis is monoclonal?

☐ **A** Karyotype analysis
☐ **B** G6PD isoenzyme analysis
☐ **C** Immunophenotyping by flow cytometry
☐ **D** Detection of immunoglobulin and T-cell receptor gene (*TCR*) rearrangements
☐ **E** All of the above

229. You have recently diagnosed a 56-year-old man with lung cancer. You are concerned about the way in which he is dealing with this bad news. Which one of the following reactions is the least likely psychological reaction to receiving a terminal diagnosis?

☐ **A** Anger
☐ **B** Anxiety
☐ **C** Confusion
☐ **D** Denial
☐ **E** Guilt

230. A 52-year old woman presents with progressive left-sided deafness over two years. On examination there is mild left limb ataxia and loss of the corneal reflex on the left. Weber's test lateralises to the right ear. What is the most likely diagnosis?

☐ **A** Presbyacusis
☐ **B** Acoustic neuroma
☐ **C** Otosclerosis
☐ **D** Ramsay-Hunt syndrome
☐ **E** Neurosarcoidosis

231. You receive funding from your local Primary Care Trust (PCT) to establish a smoking cessation clinic. You need to decide which tests you will employ to ensure that patients are indeed abstaining from smoking. Which one of the following statements regarding tobacco abstinence is false?

☐ **A** Exhaled carbon monoxide is linearly related to blood carboxyhaemoglobin
☐ **B** Blood carboxyhaemoglobin has a half-life of four hours
☐ **C** Urinary thiocyanate has a half-life of 14 days
☐ **D** Urinary cotinine has a half-life of 19 hours
☐ **E** Exhaled carbon monoxide of up to 30 ppm (parts per million) is consistent with smoking abstinence and environmental exposure

232. A 45-year-old bus driver presents with an eight-month history of increasing cough and shortness of breath associated with weight loss. The chest X-ray reveals a right apical lesion and prominent hilar lymphadenopathy. Which one of the following is the LEAST likely diagnosis in this case?

- [ ] **A** Wegener's granulomatosis
- [ ] **B** Carcinoma of the bronchus
- [ ] **C** Sarcoidosis
- [ ] **D** Non-Hodgkin's lymphoma
- [ ] **E** Tuberculosis

233. A 24-year-old woman develops symptomatic thyrotoxicosis with thyroid eye disease in the second trimester of pregnancy. What initial management would you recommend?

- [ ] **A** No treatment until she has deliverd the baby
- [ ] **B** Radioactive iodine therapy
- [ ] **C** Subtotal thyroidectomy
- [ ] **D** β-Blockers
- [ ] **E** Propylthiouracil

234. Hyperimmune immunoglobulin is NOT used in the management of which problem?

- [ ] **A** Botulism
- [ ] **B** Diphtheria
- [ ] **C** Staphylococcal toxic shock syndrome
- [ ] **D** Tetanus
- [ ] **E** Russell's pit viper envenomation

235. A 24-year-old man presents with loin pain and haematuria. He is taking no medications and examination is unremarkable. Routine investigations are normal, including a plasma creatinine of 104 μmol/l, plasma Ca²⁺ 2.42 mmol/l and uric acid 0.23 mmol/l. KUB demonstrates a single calculus in the right kidney. Which of the following statements is true?

☐ A A urine volume of less than 1 litre/day is a major risk factor for stone formation
☐ B The calculus is most likely to be composed of calcium phosphate
☐ C Identification and treatment of hypercalciuria is essential
☐ D 50% of such patients have an underlying disease contributing to stone formation
☐ E Dietary oxalate intake has no influence on stone formation

236. A 31-year-old businessman presents with a four-week history of gradual onset of rectal bleeding which accompanies bowel movements. He now describes six to ten bloody bowel movements daily, which awaken him once or twice a night, and has lost 4 kg in weight. He has no history of prior medical illness and runs six miles four times a week. He stopped smoking six months ago. On examination his temperature is 37.8 °C, blood pressure 110/70 mmHg and his pulse 90 bpm. His conjunctivae are pale. His abdomen is flat, there is tenderness in the left lower quadrant and the bowel sounds are increased. Investigations show: haemoglobin 11 g/dl, WCC 11.0 × 10⁹/l, platelets 510 × 10⁹/l; urea and electrolytes normal total bilirubin 26 μmol/l, albumin 28 g/l, alanine aminotransferase (ALT) 96 U/l, alkaline phosphatase (ALP) 110 U/l.

Stool culture shows no growth. Sigmoidoscopy reveals no perianal disease, but there is contiguous inflammation with ulceration and contact bleeding in the rectum and sigmoid. What is the most appropriate treatment for this patient?

☐ A Hospitalisation and intravenous hydrocortisone
☐ B Antibiotic therapy for presumed infection
☐ C Initial outpatient management with oral prednisolone
☐ D High-dose 5-aminosalycilate
☐ E Anti-tumour necrosis factor antibody infusion

237. **A 70-year-old woman has an elective left total knee replacement. Five days postoperatively she becomes acutely short of breath, dizzy and hypoxic, with a blood pressure of 80/40 mmHg. On examination she is cold and clammy peripherally and her ECG shows widespread T-wave inversion. What is the most important aspect of her immediate management?**

☐ A Emergency pulmonary angiography
☐ B Emergency surgical embolectomy
☐ C Intravenous heparin and transoesophageal echo with thrombolysis if proximal clot visualised
☐ D Subcutaneous low molecular weight heparin at 1.5 mg/kg once daily
☐ E Thrombolysis

238. **A 54-year-old man presents with acute onset of chest pain and breathlessness. An ECG shows ST-segment elevation in the anterior leads, consistent with a diagnosis of acute myocardial infarction. Which one of the following statements about fibrinolytic drugs is correct?**

☐ A Allergic reactions occur in around 25% of patients treated with streptokinase
☐ B Streptokinase is a protein produced by group A β-haemolytic streptococci
☐ C Repeated administration increases the effectiveness of streptokinase
☐ D Should not be used if taking warfarin therapy
☐ E Tissue plasminogen activator (t-PA) causes less bleeding than streptokinase

239. A 45-year-old lady presents with a six-week history of an expanding leg ulcer. She originally noticed a small pustule which then seemed to break down and become painful. She also suffers from ulcerative colitis, which has not been well controlled recently. On examination, there is a 5-cm ulcer on her right shin which has a raised purple edge with a necrotic centre. What is the most likely diagnosis?

- [ ] **A** Pyogenic granuloma
- [ ] **B** Venous ulcer
- [ ] **C** Erythema nodosum
- [ ] **D** Pyoderma gangrenosum
- [ ] **E** Bowen's disease

240. A 40-year-old woman presents with lethargy. She had a trans-sphenoidal resection of a non-functioning pituitary adenoma in her early thirties, followed by pituitary radiotherapy. Her current medication is thyroxine 100 μg daily and a combined oestrogen-progestogen hormone replacement therapy preparation. Which one of the following tests should be prioritised?

- [ ] **A** Short Synacthen® test
- [ ] **B** Insulin-like growth factor-1 (IGF-1)
- [ ] **C** Growth hormone stimulation test (e.g. GHRH-arginine test)
- [ ] **D** TSH
- [ ] **E** Prolactin

241. A 70-year-old woman attends the Haematology Clinic with recurrent anaemia. She has had increasing problems with anaemia since her forties. She is on long-term oral iron and needs transfusion several times a year. On examination she is generally well but is noted to have a few small red lesions on her lips and tongue. At the current clinic visit her haemoglobin 10.3 g/dl, RBC 3.37 × 10^{12}/l, MCV 72 fl, MCH 25 pg, MCHC 30 g/dl, WCC 6.5 × 10^9/l with a normal differential, platelets 375 × 10^9/l. Which one of the following is the most likely cause of her anaemia?

☐ **A** Ehlers-Danlos syndrome,
☐ **B** Immune thrombocytopenic purpura
☐ **C** Hereditary haemorrhagic telangiectasia
☐ **D** Henoch-Schönlein purpura
☐ **E** Vitamin C deficiency

242. Blood pressure is measured in a randomly selected group of 100 teenagers. The median blood pressure is 68 mmHg, mean 70 mmHg, standard deviation 7 mmHg. This information implies that the blood pressures:

☐ **A** Are normally distributed. Approximately 95% lie within the range (56–84 mmHg)
☐ **B** Are non-normally distributed. Approximately 95% lie within the range (56–84 mmHg)
☐ **C** Are normally distributed. Approximately 95% lie within the range (68.6–71.4 mmHg)
☐ **D** Are non-normally distributed. Approximately 95% lie within the range (68.6–71.4 mmHg)
☐ **E** Were not accurately measured

243. A 39-year-old man with left foot-drop comes to your clinic with a history of rhinosinusitis, cough, wheeze and fleeting shadows on his serial chest X-rays. His blood ANCA is negative. What is the most likely diagnosis?

   ☐ **A** Wegener's granulomatosis
   ☐ **B** Cystic fibrosis
   ☐ **C** Allergic bronchopulmonary aspergillosis (ABPA)
   ☐ **D** Churg-Strauss syndrome
   ☐ **E** Kartagener syndrome

244. A 45-year-old woman presents with an eight-month history of erythematous rash over the knuckles, elbows and eyelids, with no response to topical steroids. She subsequently noticed stiffness and soreness of her shoulders and proximal legs. She has weakness with difficulty lifting heavy objects or rising from a squatting position. The creatinine kinase (CK) was elevated at 5133 U/l. What is the most likely diagnosis?

   ☐ **A** Polymyositis (PM)
   ☐ **B** Fasioscapulohumeral muscular dystrophy
   ☐ **C** Dermatomyositis (DM)
   ☐ **D** Cervical myelopathy
   ☐ **E** Guillain-Barré syndrome

245. A 62-year-old man has drunk 24 units of alcohol per day for the last 15 years, and smoked heavily for 47 years. He has recently noticed difficulty walking and progressive visual disturbance. On examination he has pale optic discs. What findings are most likely on visual field examination?

   ☐ **A** Homonymous hemianopia
   ☐ **B** Centrocaecal scotoma
   ☐ **C** Peripheral field constriction
   ☐ **D** Bi-temporal hemianopia
   ☐ **E** Altitudinal field defect

246. A 27-year-old man of uncertain country of origin is brought to the Accident and Emergency Department severely unwell, with a fever, hypotension, confusion and a rapidly spreading petechial and ecchymotic rash. What is the LEAST likely diagnosis?

- [ ] **A** Meningococcal septicaemia
- [ ] **B** *Capnocytophaga canimorsus* septicaemia
- [ ] **C** Haemorrhagic smallpox
- [ ] **D** Rocky Mountain spotted fever
- [ ] **E** Staphylococcal septicaemia

247. A 45-year-old haemodialysis patient is found to have a plasma CA^{2+} of 3.15 mmol/l, parathyroid hormone (PTH) 4.2 pmol/l, phosphate 0.51 mmol/l albumin 40 g/l. He is taking perindopril 8 mg once daily, nifedipine LA 30 mg once daily, erythropoietin 2000 iu × 3 each week, aluminium hydroxide 2 caps with each meal, and alphacalcidol 250 ng three times a week. Which one of the following statements best describes this situation?

- [ ] **A** Hypercalcaemia associated with osteodystrophy responds to high-dose oral steroids
- [ ] **B** Secondary hyperparathyroidism is treated with the 1-alpha-hydroxylated form of vitamin D
- [ ] **C** Renal osteomalacia will respond to the 25-hydroxylated form of Vitamin D
- [ ] **D** Tertiary hyperparathyroidism always requires parathyroidectomy
- [ ] **E** The course of osteodystrophy is not altered by transplantation

248. A characteristic feature of fundoscopy in infective endocarditis is

- [ ] **A** Hard exudates
- [ ] **B** Optic atrophy
- [ ] **C** Papilloedema
- [ ] **D** Roth spots
- [ ] **E** Silver wiring

249. A 68-year-old hypertensive man presents with chest pain of sudden onset. In the ambulance he becomes progressively more hypotensive. On admission, pain is continuing, pulse is 140 bpm, blood pressure 120/60 mmHg, his JVP is raised at 6 cm and rises further with inspiration. His ECG shows ST elevation in II, AVF and III. Which one of the following is most likely to represent the diagnosis?

- [ ] **A** Kawasaki disease
- [ ] **B** Massive pulmonary embolism
- [ ] **C** Posterior myocardial infarction
- [ ] **D** Type 1 aortic dissection
- [ ] **E** Viral pericarditis

250. A 67-year-old man with atrial fibrillation and cardiac failure is treated with digoxin. The dose of his medication was increased recently, and shortly afterwards he developed nausea, vomiting, palpitations and hypotension. On admission to hospital, plasma digoxin concentration was found to be 3 μg/l (normal range 1–2 μg/l) and digoxin toxicity is thought to account for his deterioration. Which one of the following is the most important early step in his management?

- [ ] **A** Acute bolus administration of intravenous lidocaine (lignocaine)
- [ ] **B** Administration of loop diuretic to enhance drug clearance
- [ ] **C** Correction of fluid and electrolyte abnormalities
- [ ] **D** Intravenous administration of calcium gluconate
- [ ] **E** Urgent haemodialysis

251. A 30-year-old man with type 1 diabetes attends his 'annual review' appointment. Dipstick urinalysis in the clinic is positive for glucose, but negative for blood and protein. His blood pressure is 140/80 mmHg. Laboratory results include an elevated albumin:creatinine ratio (in a mid-stream urine specimen) and a serum creatinine of 90 μmol/l. A subsequent early-morning urine specimen confirms the elevated albumin:creatinine ratio. Which one of the following should be prioritised in his management?

☐ **A** Measure urinary albumin excretion every year
☐ **B** Start him on an ACE inhibitor (ACEI)
☐ **C** Renal ultrasound
☐ **D** Mid-stream urine specimen for microscopy and culture
☐ **E** Autoimmune profile

252. A nine-month-old boy of Ghanaian origin, born in Dublin, Ireland, is taken to his General Practitioner because he has been upset and crying for two days. On examination the only abnormality is swelling and tenderness of the fingers of his left hand. The GP orders blood tests and an X-ray. There is no abnormality on X-ray of the hand. His haemoglobin is 7.5 g/dl, MCV 103 fl, MCH 33pg, MCHC 32.5 g/dl, WCC 13.3 × 10⁹/l with a neutrophil leucocytosis, platelets 175 × 10⁹/l reticulocytes 185 × 10⁹/l (normal range 50–100 × 10⁹/l), urea 3.5 mmol/l, Na⁺ 138 mmol/l, K⁺ 3.8 mmol/l, creatinine 65 μmol/l, AST 30 U/l, ALT 59 U/l, ALP 48 U/l, bilirubin 47 μmol/l, LDH 1128 U/l. Which one of the following is the most likely cause of this baby's problem?

☐ **A** Sickle cell anaemia
☐ **B** Juvenile chronic arthritis
☐ **C** β-Thalassaemia major
☐ **D** Congenital sideroblastic anaemia
☐ **E** Fanconi's anaemia

253. A 57-year-old man presents with numbness in the legs and unsteadiness. On examination there is bilateral nystagmus and there is marked ataxia. Sensation to pinprick is impaired bilaterally in the lower limbs, and reflexes are generally depressed, with flexor plantars. Routine biochemical and haematological studies are normal, as are a CT scan of the head and routine CSF examination. Four months later he is unable to walk and has developed progressive cognitive impairment. An MRI scan shows cerebellar atrophy and diffuse white matter lesions. What is the most likely diagnosis?

- [ ] **A** Paraneoplastic syndrome
- [ ] **B** Acute disseminated encephalomyelitis
- [ ] **C** Spinocerebellar ataxia
- [ ] **D** Creutzfeldt-Jakob disease
- [ ] **E** Wilson's disease

254. A 47-year-old man with polymyositis develops progressive dyspnoea and a cough over 12 to 18 months. He has some patchy shadowing at both lung bases. Which one of the following statements is true concerning interstitial lung disease (ILD) in polymyositis?

- [ ] **A** Severity of lung disease has a positive correlation with myositis severity
- [ ] **B** Is associated with organising pneumonia
- [ ] **C** Is more common with elevated creatine kinase (CK)
- [ ] **D** Gas transfer factor (TLCO) is supranormal because of co-existent respiratory muscle weakness.
- [ ] **E** Has a negative correlation with the presence of t-RNA synthetases

255. Four patients on a ward develop acute diarrhoea and vomiting associated with fever. Within 48 hours a number of staff and other patients have also developed the illness. What is the likely causative agent?

- [ ] **A** *Salmonella enteritidis*
- [ ] **B** Staphylococcal enterotoxin
- [ ] **C** *Clostridium difficile*
- [ ] **D** Enterovirus
- [ ] **E** Norovirus

256. A 76-year-old farmer is known to have rheumatoid arthritis affecting the hands, both knees and the right shoulder. He presents to the hospital with fever, chills, and painful swelling of the left knee. His symptoms began the day before and worsened to the point that he now cannot walk. He has no history of recent trauma or a fall. His temperature is 39 °C. His disease was well controlled with oral NSAIDs, prednisolone 5 mg orally and methotrexate 10 mg weekly. At this point, which one of the following actions is the most appropriate in the management of his illness?

- [ ] **A** Aspirate the synovial fluid from the left knee
- [ ] **B** Double the steroid dose
- [ ] **C** Order radiographs of the left knee
- [ ] **D** Increase the methotrexate dose to 15 mg weekly
- [ ] **E** Arrange for full blood count and ESR

257. A 55-year-old man with a prior anterior myocardial infarction has developed increasing shortness of breath on exertion. He is now breathless on climbing one flight of stairs or walking 50 m on the flat. He does not suffer with orthopnoea. An echocardiogram shows an akinetic anterior wall with severely impaired left ventricular systolic function. Which pharmacological treatments are most likely to improve his prognosis?

- [ ] **A** ACE inhibitor, angiotensin-II blocker, β-blocker
- [ ] **B** ACE inhibitor, angiotensin-II blocker, spironolactone
- [ ] **C** Amiodarone, β-blocker, ACE inhibitor
- [ ] **D** β-Blocker, ACE inhibitor, spironolactone
- [ ] **E** β-Blocker, angiotensin-II blocker, spironolactone

258. A 68-year-old patient with diabetic nephropathy and mild impairment of excretory renal function develops diarrhoea and vomiting and is found by her GP to have an *Escherichia coli* urinary tract infection. She is prescribed ciprofloxacin but 24 hours later she presents in acute renal failure. Her pulse is 78 bpm, blood pressure 112/68 mmHg lying, falling to 98/60 mmHg on standing, temperature 37.6 °C. Abdominal examination is unremarkable. What is the most likely diagnosis?

- [ ] **A** Acute tubular necrosis
- [ ] **B** Pyelonephritis
- [ ] **C** Interstitial nephritis
- [ ] **D** Intraglomerular thrombi
- [ ] **E** Post-infectious glomerulonephritis

259. A 34-year-old woman has been receiving antibiotic treatment for an uncomplicated lower urinary tract infection for four days. She has now developed jaundice, and serum biochemistry shows bilirubin 36 μmol/l, GTT 384 U/l, ALT 44 U/l and ALP 298 U/l. Which one of the following antibiotics is most likely to have accounted for these abnormalities?

- [ ] **A** Amoxicillin
- [ ] **B** Ciprofloxacin
- [ ] **C** Co-amoxiclav
- [ ] **D** Flucloxacillin
- [ ] **E** Nitrofurantoin

260. A 42-year-old woman with a history of heavy alcohol intake for the past 15 years presents with constant abdominal pain radiating to the back, loose motions and a 20-kg weight loss over the past year. Investigations: haemoglobin 11 g/dl, MCV 110 fl, red cell folate 360 µg/l, serum vitamin B_{12} 60 pmol/l, urea and electrolytes normal, plasma glucose 13 mmol/l, total bilirubin 10 µmol/l, albumin 28 g/l, ALT 36 U/l, ALP 180 U/l, corrected calcium 2.0 mmol/l. Stool examination: fat globules. Ultrasound abdomen reveals hyperechoic liver (pancreas not visualised). In this patient:

☐ A Plain X-ray of the abdomen is the most sensitive test to demonstrate pancreatic calcification

☐ B Steatorrhoea is related to deficiency of chymotrypsin

☐ C B_{12} deficiency is related to deficiency of pancreatic amylase

☐ D Hypocalcaemia is related to fat malabsorption

☐ E Abnormality in the D-xylose test is diagnostic of pancreatic exocrine deficiency

261. A 50-year-old menopausal woman consults her GP about hormone replacement therapy (HRT). She has brought a list of the benefits of HRT that she found on the Internet: which one is LEAST supported by the available evidence?

☐ A Treatment of hot flushes

☐ B Prevention of hip fractures

☐ C Prevention of ischaemic heart disease

☐ D Treatment of vaginal dryness

☐ E Prevention of vertebral crush fractures

262. A 56-year-old man with type 2 diabetes presents with right-sided foot-drop immediately after tripping and falling over while playing golf. On examination there is weakness of dorsiflexion, inversion and eversion of the right foot. There is no sensory disturbance. Which structure is most likely to have been damaged?

☐ A Sciatic nerve

☐ B L5 nerve root

☐ C Tibial nerve

☐ D Femoral nerve

☐ E Common peroneal nerve

263. A 40-year-old man presents with a six-month history of night sweats and weight loss. On examination he has cervical and inguinal lymphadenopathy. Biopsy of a cervical gland shows a lymphoid infiltrate with scattered Reed-Sternberg cells which is classified as mixed-cellularity Hodgkin's disease. CT scan of his chest and abdomen shows widespread para-aortic lymphadenopathy and a normal-sized liver and spleen. His haemoglobin is 13.5 g/dl, WCC 14.5 × 10^9/l with a neutrophil leucocytosis, platelets 438 × 10^9/l, and a bone marrow aspirate and trephine do not show any involvement with Hodgkin's disease. What stage is his Hodgkin's disease?

- [ ] **A** Stage IVA
- [ ] **B** Stage IA
- [ ] **C** Stage IIIB
- [ ] **D** Stage IIIA
- [ ] **E** Stage IIB

264. A 29-year-old woman gives birth at 36 weeks of pregnancy to a baby with a hypoplastic left eye. Which event in the mother during the first trimester of pregnancy is likely to be responsible?

- [ ] **A** Chickenpox
- [ ] **B** Secondary syphilis
- [ ] **C** Rubella vaccination
- [ ] **D** Cytomegalovirus (CMV) reactivation
- [ ] **E** Acute parvovirus B19 infection

265. A 52-year-old woman presents with headache, weakness and confusion. Getting little history from the patient, you request a number of investigations. Your new House Officer takes some arterial blood gases despite you having told him not to bother as her oxygen saturation is normal at 97% by pulse oximetry while breathing room air. The PaO_2 is 8.5 kPa (65 mmHg). Which one of the following is the most likely explanation?

- [ ] **A** Cerebrovascular accident with aspiration pneumonia
- [ ] **B** Venous sample taken by House Officer
- [ ] **C** Guillain-Barré syndrome
- [ ] **D** Carbon monoxide poisoning
- [ ] **E** Subarachnoid haemorrhage

266. Which one of the following bone disorders is associated with defective osteoclast function, leading to obliteration of the medullary cavity in all the bones?

☐ **A** Paget's disease
☐ **B** Osteoporosis
☐ **C** Osteomalacia
☐ **D** Osteogenesis imperfecta
☐ **E** Osteopetrosis

267. A 45-year-old man is admitted with acute renal failure. His creatinine is 1564 μmol/l and his urea is 76 mmol/l. His blood pressure is 200/110 mmHg, he is oliguric and he has pulmonary oedema confirmed on chest X-ray. He is given a bolus of 200 mg phenytoin intravenously and is urgently commenced on haemodialysis via a central venous catheter, with a target weight loss of 1.5 kg. One hour into dialysis he begins to complain of chest pain. Shortly afterwards he becomes confused and disorientated. His blood pressure is 180/100 mmHg. What is the most likely explanation?

☐ **A** Air embolism
☐ **B** Dysequilibrium syndrome
☐ **C** Intravascular volume contraction
☐ **D** Pericardial tamponade
☐ **E** Pneumothorax

268. A 28-year-old man has been referred to the clinic for investigations after returning from a backpacking holiday in the Far East. He has history of jaundice nine months ago, when he was told he had 'hepatitis'. His symptoms resolved over a few weeks then and he is now asymptomatic. On investigation he is found to be positive for hepatitis B surface antigen. What advice is the most appropriate to give?

- [ ] A It is too early to expect clearance of hepatitis
- [ ] B He could transmit hepatitis B to his partner if he is hepatitis Be antigen-positive
- [ ] C He would be considered an inactive carrier if he is hepatitis Be antigen-negative
- [ ] D Liver biopsy is indicated in all those with hepatitis B surface antigen, irrespective of other investigation results
- [ ] E He would need antiviral therapy irrespective of other investigation results

269. A 40-year-old woman patient presents with increasing shortness on breath on exertion and peripheral oedema. On examination her pulse is 80 bpm and blood pressure 140/70 mmHg. Her JVP is raised and rises further on inspiration; auscultation reveals a gallop rhythm. A chest X-ray shows a normal-sized heart, some upper-lobe blood diversion and mild pulmonary oedema, and marked osteopenia. Routine bloods show: haemoglobin 9.0 g/dl, WCC 8.2×10^9/l, platelets 170×10^9/l, ESR 80 mm/h, Na$^+$ 139 mmol/l, K$^+$4.1 mmol/l, creatine 160 μmol/l, Ca^{2+} 2.65 mmol/l, albumin 15 g/l, total protein 67 g/l.

ECG shows septal Q waves. Echocardiography shows no pericardial fluid, and a stiff ventricle of normal dimensions. Dipstick urinalysis shows protein $+ + +$. What is this lady's cardiac abnormality most likely to represent?

- [ ] A Constrictive pericardial disease
- [ ] B Dilated cardiomyopathy
- [ ] C Hypertensive heart disease
- [ ] D Ischaemic ventricular impairment
- [ ] E Restrictive myocardial disease

270. A 42-year-old woman has had asthma for several years, treated with intermittent inhaled salbutamol for symptomatic relief. She is admitted to Casualty with a severe attack that has persisted for one hour, despite administration of her inhaler. Which one of the following drugs is likely to be of greatest immediate benefit in her acute management?

- [ ] **A** Intravenous aminophylline infusion
- [ ] **B** Intravenous broad-spectrum antibiotics
- [ ] **C** Intravenous hydrocortisone
- [ ] **D** Nebulised ipratropium bromide
- [ ] **E** Nebulised salbutamol

271. A previously healthy 27-year-old man presents complaining of the sudden onset of a severe headache and neck pain shortly after showering. On examination you find a right homonymous hemianopia but no other focal neurological signs. What is the most likely diagnosis?

- [ ] **A** Vertebral artery dissection
- [ ] **B** Paradoxical embolism
- [ ] **C** Multiple sclerosis
- [ ] **D** Cerebral vasculitis
- [ ] **E** CNS lymphoma

272. A 50-year-old intravenous drug user develops a slowly progressive vasculitic rash with palpable purpura on his feet, arthralgia and peripheral neuropathy. He is found to have proteinuria, haematuria and hypertension. A renal biopsy shows a membranoproliferative glomerulonephritis. What is the most likely cause?

- [ ] **A** HIV-associated nephropathy
- [ ] **B** Chronic hepatitis B
- [ ] **C** Chronic hepatitis C
- [ ] **D** *Staphylcoccus aureus* endocarditis of the tricuspid valve
- [ ] **E** Post-streptococcal glomerulonephritis

273. A 64-year-old man has suffered from recurrent episodes of acute gout. His General Practitioner has prescribed allopurinol 100 mg daily. Which one of the following statements regarding the pharmacological effects of allopurinol is correct?

- [ ] **A** Acute gout is a recognised adverse effect
- [ ] **B** Combination with non-steroidal anti-inflammatory drugs is often hazardous
- [ ] **C** Increases renal tubular secretion of urate
- [ ] **D** Reduces the effectiveness of warfarin
- [ ] **E** Should not be used in asymptomatic hyperuricaemia

274. A 65-year-old woman is found to have temporal arteritis and is started on high-dose steroids. Her GP is aware of the need to protect her from osteoporosis, but is unsure which agent to use. Which one of the following is most appropriate to prevent the patient suffering osteoporotic fractures during her steroid treatment?

- [ ] **A** Alendronate
- [ ] **B** Fluoride supplements
- [ ] **C** Cyclical etidronate (Didronel PMO®)
- [ ] **D** Calcium and vitamin D supplements (Calcichew® D3 Forte)
- [ ] **E** Hormone replacement therapy

275. At an antenatal booking clinic a 24-year-old primigravida is found to have dipstick proteinuria and a blood pressure of 156/84 mmHg. Creatinine is found to be 78 μmol/l and 24-hour urinary protein excretion 1.2 g. Blood pressure is controlled with methyldopa 250 mg tds and the pregnancy proceeds to term. Three months after delivery proteinuria persists. An ultrasound scan demonstrates that both kidneys are of normal size and unobstructed but suggests a 'scar' at the upper pole of the right kidney. Intravenous urography confirms focal scarring at the upper pole of the right kidney with underlying calyceal clubbing. Which of the following best describes the situation?

☐ A Renal biopsy should be performed
☐ B The scar is likely to have formed before the age of ten years
☐ C Urinary tract infection plays no part in the pathogenesis of this disease
☐ D There is a 5% chance of the patient's offspring developing renal failure
☐ E The presence of proteinuria is of no prognostic significance

276. A 29-year-old woman who has recently returned from Thailand presents with right upper abdominal pain of two weeks' duration, associated with anorexia. She has had fever for the past four days' associated with rigors on the last two days. On examination she is febrile, looks pale and has tender liver, palpable 5 cm below the costal margin. There are no other stigmata of chronic liver disease. Investigations: haemoglobin: 12 g/dl, WCC 16.4 × 10⁹/l, platelets 502 × 10⁹/l, urea and electrolytes normal, total bilirubin 11 μmol/l, albumin 29 g/l, ALT 98 U/l, ALP 208 U/l. Which one of the following statements is true when the diagnosis of amoebic liver abscess is suspected?

☐ A Absence of a history of dysentery excludes the diagnosis
☐ B Stool examination would demonstrate tropozoites of *Entamoeba histolytica* in 75% of cases
☐ C Isotope liver scan would be the imaging modality of choice
☐ D Serology for *E. histolytica* is positive in > 90% of cases
☐ E Treatment with metronidazole is effective in eradicating *E. histolytica*

277. A 12-year-old girl has been diagnosed with asthma, and has been prescribed regular disodium cromoglicate. Which one of the following statements best describes its pharmacological properties?

☐ A Acts by stimulating mast cell degranulation
☐ B Is effective in acute asthma if administered early
☐ C Can be administered as an inhaled powder or aerosol or nebulised solution
☐ D Does not prevent exercise-induced asthma
☐ E Should not be used in combination with salbutamol

278. A 78-year-old farmer presents with a two-week history of haematuria and extensive bruising. He has been previously fit and active with no history of bleeding disorder or other illness. He is not on any medication. On examination he has extensive bruising on his legs and buttocks. There is nothing else of note. On investigation his results are: haemoglobin 8.5 g/dl, WCC 10.5 × 10⁹/l, platelets 215 × 10⁹/l, prothrombin time 16 s (normal range 12–17 s), APTT 57 s (normal range 24–38 s), thrombin time 18 s (normal range 14–22 s), fibrinogen 2.6 g/l (normal range 2–5 g/l). Which one of the following is the most likely cause of his bleeding disorder?

☐ A Haemophilia A
☐ B Accidental warfarin overdose
☐ C Haemophilia B
☐ D Acquired haemophilia
☐ E Excess heparin

279. A 33-year-old woman on the oral contraceptive pill has just returned from Australia where she had a climbing accident and broke both her legs, which are in full-length plaster. You see her in the Accident and Emergency Department with several symptoms that make you suspicious of pulmonary embolism (PE). Which one of the following is the most likely symptom she will have if your diagnosis is correct?

☐ A Dyspnoea
☐ B Pleuritic chest pain
☐ C Cough
☐ D Haemoptysis
☐ E Leg swelling

280. A 42-year-old woman with rheumatoid arthritis (RA), previously well controlled with sulfasalazine, presents with deep red, necrotic ulcers with undermined, violaceous, oedematous borders. The ulcers are 10 × 5 cm in diameter, covering the anterior border of the right leg. Trials with systemic and local steroid therapy over the last two-months did not help to improve the ulcers. Which one of the following is the most likely diagnosis?

☐ A Ulcerated rheumatoid nodule
☐ B Erythema nodosum
☐ C Pyoderma gangrenosum
☐ D Fixed drug rash
☐ E Vasculitic skin rash

281. A 50-year-old woman who had a liver transplantation three months ago for cirrhosis secondary to autoimmune hepatitis visits her General Practitioner for prescriptions. She is on a combination of ciclosporin, azathioprine and prednisolone. Which of the following most accurately describes the mechanism of action of her medication?

☐ A The immunosuppressive effect of ciclosporin is due to inhibition of transforming growth factor-β (TGF-β)
☐ B Prednisolone acts on the receptors on the cell surface
☐ C Azathioprine inhibits pyrimidine synthesis
☐ D Ciclosporin is associated with less hirsutism than tacrolimus
☐ E Mycophenolate mofetil acts more selectively on lymphocytes

282. A 48-year-old man presents to the Accident and Emergency Department with difficulty walking, which has progressed over a period of six weeks. He has no back pain but has noticed disturbance of sensation in both legs. On examination he has pyramidal weakness of his left leg, with exaggerated reflexes and an upgoing plantar on that side. Joint-position sense is impaired at the right big toe. There are no other signs. What is the most likely diagnosis?

☐ A Lumbosacral disc prolapse
☐ B Syringomyelia
☐ C Guillain-Barré syndrome
☐ D Brown-Séquard syndrome
☐ E Anterior spinal artery occlusion

283. A 43-year-old woman presents with breathlessness, increasing over the last year, and malaise over the last two months. She has an exercise tolerance of half a mile but suffers with marked orthopnoea when she lies on her back, though this is relieved by lying on the right side. On examination she has a widespread vasculitic rash and a mid-diastolic murmur. Which one of the following is most likely to represent the diagnosis?

☐ A Infective endocarditis
☐ B Left atrial myxoma
☐ C Mitral stenosis
☐ D Sinus of Valsalva aneurysm
☐ E Tricuspid stenosis

284. A 45-year-old woman who has lived in Mexico City for the previous year develops a swinging fever and right shoulder-tip pain. An abdominal ultrasound shows a single, echo-poor area, $5 \times 6 \times 8$ cm in size, in the right lobe of the liver, consistent with a cyst or abscess with no obvious septa. The blood neutrophil count is $17 \times 10^9/l$, eosinophil count $0.4 \times 10^9/l$. What is the likely diagnosis?

☐ A *Streptococcus milleri (anginosus)*-group liver abscess
☐ B Amoebic liver abscess
☐ C Hepatic cysticercosis
☐ D Hepatic hydatid disease
☐ E Hepatic actinomycosis

285. Certain drugs are known to reduce the effectiveness of the combined oral contraceptive pill (COCP) and can result in unintended pregnancy. Which one of the following is NOT a recognised cause of reduced COCP effectiveness?

- [ ] **A** Allopurinol
- [ ] **B** Carbamazepine
- [ ] **C** Griseofulvin
- [ ] **D** Phenytoin
- [ ] **E** Rifampicin

286. A 45-year-old man presents with symptoms of polyuria and polydipsia. A random capillary glucose concentration is 20 mmol/l. His GP is a little uncomfortable about some features of his presentation, which do not seem typical of type 2 diabetes. He therefore telephones the local Diabetes Centre to ask if the patient should start insulin treatment immediately. Which one of the following is most suggestive that the patient has type 1 diabetes?

- [ ] **A** One plus of ketonuria on dipstick urinalysis
- [ ] **B** A history of weight loss of half a stone over the previous few months
- [ ] **C** No family history of diabetes
- [ ] **D** A venous bicarbonate concentration of 8 mmol/l
- [ ] **E** Blood pressure of 130/74 mmHg

287. A 24-year-old homosexual man presents with ankle swelling. Dipstick urinalysis demonstrates proteinuria +++ and no blood. Creatinine is 125 μmol/l and plasma albumin 22 g/l. 24-hour urine protein excretion is 6 g. He is known to be HIV-positive, with a viral load of 180,000 copies/ml and a CD4 count of 380 cells/μl. Blood pressure is 128/64 mmHg. He is otherwise well and has no history of any AIDS-defining illness. He has not received antiretroviral chemotherapy. Ultrasound scan demonstrates large echogenic kidneys. What is renal biopsy most likely to show?

- [ ] **A** Minimal change nephropathy
- [ ] **B** Acute tubular necrosis
- [ ] **C** Focal segmental glomerulosclerosis
- [ ] **D** Membranous glomerulonephropathy
- [ ] **E** IgA nephropathy

MRCP1: 300 BEST OF FIVE QUESTIONS

288. A 58-year-old man presents with abdominal distension and weight loss of two months' duration. He has no past history of jaundice, but admits intravenous drug abuse in his twenties. He had jaundice 35 years ago and was told he had 'hepatitis', which resolved. On examination he has muscle wasting, jaundice, hepatosplenomegaly and ascites. Investigations show: haemoglobin 10.9 g/dl, WCC 3.2 × 10⁹/l, platelets 64 × 10⁹/l, total bilirubin 77 μmol/l, albumin 24 g/l, ALT 99 U/l, ALP 180 U/l, anti-HBc-positive, HBs Ag-negative, hepatitis C antibody- and RNA-positive. Which one of the following statements is true with regards to this patient?

- [ ] **A** Diagnosis of cirrhosis secondary to chronic hepatitis B is likely
- [ ] **B** Hepatocellular carcinoma needs to be excluded
- [ ] **C** He is a good candidate for antiviral therapy
- [ ] **D** Past hepatitis B infection does not affect hepatitis C-related liver disease
- [ ] **E** Hepatitis C infection does not recur after transplantation if he abstains from intravenous drug abuse

289. A 74-year-old man attends the Outpatient Department for investigation of recent falls. He is found to have increased tone and rigidity in his upper and lower limbs, and a paucity of facial expression. You suspect a diagnosis of Parkinson's disease. Which ONE of the following would be the most appropriate initial treatment?

- [ ] **A** Apomorphine
- [ ] **B** Trihexyphenidyl (benzhexol)
- [ ] **C** Co-careldopa
- [ ] **D** Levodopa
- [ ] **E** Selegiline

290. A 26-year-old man has a bone marrow transplant from his HLA-identical 20-year-old sister for acute myeloid leukaemia in second remission. On day 20 post-transplant he develops a rash on his hands and feet. At this time his haemoglobin is 10.7 g/dl, WCC 3.2 × 10⁹/l, platelets 20 × 10⁹/l. On day 21 he experiences vomiting ten times per day and diarrhoea of 2l/day. His temperature is constantly 37.8 °C despite broad-spectrum antibiotics. His investigations on day 21 show: urea 9.5 mmol/l, Na⁺ 145 mmol/l, K⁺ 3.0 mmol/l, creatinine 154 μmol/l, AST 56 U/l, ALT 69 U/l, ALP 254 U/l, bilirubin 35 μmol/l, LDH 879 U/l. Which one of the following is the most likely cause of his symptoms?

- A Graft-versus-host disease
- B Rotavirus infection
- C Gastroenteritis
- D Relapse of acute myeloid leukaemia
- E Graft failure

291. A 58-year-old man presents with progressive breathlessness. Chest X-ray shows interstitial shadowing. He smokes 20 cigarettes per day. Which one of the following is the least likely diagnosis?

- A Extrinsic allergic alveolitis (EAA)
- B Langerhans cell histiocytosis (LCH)
- C Desquamative interstitial pneumonitis (DIP)
- D Respiratory bronchiolitis interstitial lung disease (RB-ILD)
- E Cryptogenic fibrosing alveolitis (CFA)

292. A 48-year-old woman consults her doctor because of a two-year history of excessive fatigue and easy tiredness. She reports non-specific joint pain around the elbows and knees with early morning stiffness lasting two hours. The patient also reports that she takes frequent sips of water when eating and could not wear contact lenses because they were uncomfortable. She is not on any medications and the past medical history is unremarkable. Examination revealed red eyes and mild tenderness at the joint lines in both knees but no active synovitis. The ESR was elevated at 78 mm/h and the rheumatoid factor was positive at 1/1024. What is the most likely diagnosis?

☐ A Fibromyalgia
☐ B Polymyalgia rheumatica
☐ C Systemic lupus erythematosus
☐ D Sjögren's syndrome
☐ E Rheumatoid arthritis

293. A 43-year-old man is taking omeprazole 20 mg daily to treat reflux oesophagitis. He is symptom-free and has not noticed any side effects. Which one of the following is recognised as a characteristic effect of regular omeprazole treatment?

☐ A 80–85% reduction in gastric acid secretion
☐ B Constipation
☐ C Increased absorption of ferrous sulphate
☐ D Increased risk of gastric carcinoma
☐ E Increased risk of *Salmonella* gastroenteritis

294. A 34-year-old schoolteacher presents with a two-month history of swelling and discomfort in the right knee and the left ankle. She walks with a limp. The patient's past history significantly revealed recurrent episodes of bilateral uveitis over the past ten years, treated with topical corticosteroids. She was referred for further assessment. Which one of the following disorders is the least likely cause of this patient's illness?

- [ ] **A** Psoriatic arthritis
- [ ] **B** Rheumatoid arthritis (RA)
- [ ] **C** Behçet's disease
- [ ] **D** Sarcoidosis
- [ ] **E** Syphilis

295. A new drug is being developed for the treatment of depression. Animal models have shown that it reduces markers of anxiety, and preclinical tests have not found any toxicity. When the drug is first administered to humans, which one of the following is the most appropriate clinical trial design?

- [ ] **A** Comparison with licensed drug in healthy volunteers
- [ ] **B** Comparison with licensed drug in patients with depression
- [ ] **C** Open-label placebo-controlled trial in healthy volunteers
- [ ] **D** Open-label non-controlled study in patients with depression
- [ ] **E** Randomised placebo-controlled trial in healthy volunteers

296. A 37-year-old woman is diagnosed with HIV infection. In accordance with local protocols, you commence treatment with a combination of several antiretroviral drugs. Which one of the following adverse effects is NOT a recognised feature of the appropriate antiretroviral agent?

- [ ] **A** Acute pancreatitis and didanosine (DDI)
- [ ] **B** Peripheral neuropathy and lamivudine (3TC)
- [ ] **C** Gingival hyperplasia and zidovudine (AZT)
- [ ] **D** Deranged liver biochemistry and stavudine (d4T)
- [ ] **E** Myalgia and zalcitabine (DDC)

297. Which one of the following pharmacological abnormalities is a characteristic finding in patients with impaired hepatic function?

☐ **A** Increased first-pass metabolism
☐ **B** Increased protein binding
☐ **C** Reduced bioavailability
☐ **D** Reduced effectiveness of diuretic treatment
☐ **E** Reduced effectiveness of warfarin

298. A 60-year-old man presents 24 hours after an episode of chest pain at rest, associated with lateral T-wave changes and a positive troponin I. His random cholesterol the morning after admission is 6.2 mmol/l. What is the most appropriate management with respect to his lipids?

☐ **A** Dietary advice
☐ **B** Commence simvastatin
☐ **C** Perform fasting lipid sample
☐ **D** Recheck cholesterol in six weeks
☐ **E** Request HDL/IDL ratio

299. A 40-year-old man with a body mass index of 32 (normal range 22–26) is found to have a blood pressure of 160/90 mmHg. He is recalled for a further blood pressure check two weeks later when he has a blood pressure of 146/87 mmHg. He drinks 50 units of alcohol per week but does not smoke. What is the most appropriate management?

☐ **A** Atenolol
☐ **B** Bendroflumethiazide (bendrofluazide)
☐ **C** Lifestyle advice and recheck blood pressure in six months
☐ **D** No action required
☐ **E** Ramipril

300. A 30-year-old woman experiences a brief episode of left hemiparesis, with complete resolution after a few minutes. A similar episode occurs a few weeks later. She has no other medical problems and has no risk factors for vascular disease. A transthoracic echocardiogram is normal. What is the most likely reason for her symptoms?

- ☐ **A** Carotid stenosis
- ☐ **B** Atrial fibrillation
- ☐ **C** Patent foramen ovale
- ☐ **D** Pulmonary embolism
- ☐ **E** Subarachnoid haemorrhage

Answers

1. **D: Ramipril, simvastatin, aspirin, atenolol**
   A wealth of end-point data supports statins in both primary and secondary prevention of athersclerotic disease. Fibrates are effective in lowering LDL cholesterol and triglycerides but do not have sufficient mortality data to compete with statins. Clopidogrel may be used in addition to aspirin or as second-line antiplatelet therapy. Warfarin should replace aspirin only if there is a specific indication. ACE inhibition is preferred to angiotensin blockade.

2. **E: Polycystic ovarian syndrome**
   Clues to the diagnosis of polycystic ovarian syndrome (PCOS) include the fact that her periods have 'always' been irregular, and that she is a little overweight and a little hirsute, but not virilised. PCOS is also common, and the question asks about the most 'likely' diagnosis in a patient in a primary care setting.

3. **B: Temporal lobe uncus across the tentorium**
   Space-occupying lesions can impair consciousness either through direct extension of the lesion into the midbrain and brainstem or, more commonly, by lateral and downward displacement of these structures, with or without herniation of the medial part of the temporal lobe through the tentorium. This lateral displacement typically crushes the upper midbrain against the opposite free edge of the tentorium, causing an upgoing plantar ipsilateral to the hemispheric lesions. All forms of brainstem herniation can cause depression of respiration, extensor posturing and bilateral upgoing plantars. The uncal syndrome differs mainly in that early drowsiness is accompanied or preceded by unilateral pupillary dilatation, often (but not always) due to compression of the oculomotor nerve by the herniated uncus.

4. **A: Extent of protein binding**
   Bioavailability represents the extent of systemic drug absorption, calculated as the percentage of area under the concentration-time curve during oral administration, compared to intravenous administration ($AUC_{oral}/AUC_{iv} \times 100$). Formulation is important: suspensions tend to have greater bioavailability than capsules, which in turn have better bioavailability than tablets. Drug metabolism by the liver and gastrointestinal mucosa both influence bioavailability. For drugs with extensive first-pass metabolism, impaired liver function can increase bioavailability. The rate of gastrointestinal emptying determines the time allowed for drug dissolution and absorption. Drugs that are susceptible to hydrolysis, e.g. lidocaine (lignocaine), tend to have low bioavailability.

5.   **D: Henoch-Schönlein purpura**
Henoch-Schönlein purpura is the most likely diagnosis. It is characterised by a purpuric rash most prominent in the lower legs and buttocks, and affecting the extensor surfaces of the limbs. It is associated with arthralgia, arthritis, gastrointestinal symptoms and renal involvement (nephritis). There may be a history of preceding streptococcal infection. A raised serum IgA or its deposition in the skin is regarded by some as diagnostic. The histological process is a leucocytoclastic vasculitis. Pigmented purpuric dermatosis is a capillaritis causing non-palpable purpura and haemosiderin deposition, typically in the lower limbs, without systemic symptoms. Linear IgA disease presents with erythematous blisters, often with mucosal and conjunctival involvement. Erythema multiforme is a erythematous vesiculobullous disorder with a variety of causes. Erythema marginatum is the typical skin manifestation of rheumatic fever, and is an asymptomatic, pinkish eruption appearing in semi circles or rings.

6.   **D: Anaemia of chronic disease**
This occurs in patients with chronic inflammatory or malignant disease. This lady had rheumatoid arthritis. It is characterised by:
   • A normochromic or mildly hypochromic, normocytic anaemia
   • Reduced serum iron and TIBC
   • Serum ferritin normal or raised
   • Normal bone marrow iron stores but reduced iron in erythroid cells

7.   **C: Herpes simplex virus (HSV) type 1**
The history, CSF and MRI findings are typical for HSV encephalitis. CT of the head may not show any abnormality. (An MRI scan may also be normal in the early stages.) The findings, apart from the MRI scan, would fit with disseminated Lyme disease and secondary syphilis, although encephalitis is not frequently seen in the UK. *Listeria* meningitis remains uncommon in the UK, but is more common in the elderly. Most patients with *Listeria* meningitis will have a neutrophilic CSF. *Listeria* can also cause a brainstem encephalitis (rhombencephalitis) with a similar prodrome and CSF findings, but this usually progresses with cranial nerve signs and changes in the brainstem seen on MRI. TB meningitis can also present in a similar fashion, apart from the MRI findings, although the CSF protein is usually much higher.

8. B: These features are consistent with preproliferative diabetic retinopathy

Progression of retinopathy during pregnancy is common, but the patient does not require treatment at this stage. Monthly review would be reasonable.

9. A: The voice is located in subjective space

Pseudohallucinations are perceptions experienced in the mind and not in the external environment. They are not, however, subject to conscious control. They are not pathognomonic of any condition and can be associated with grieving. Whether the voice is of a real person or in the second or third person is not relevant to the definition of a pseudohallucination.

10. E: Intravenous normal saline to maintain a CVP of 6–10 cmH_2O

Approximately 4% of patients develop hyponatraemia postoperatively. This is particularly common following relief of obstruction, when polyuria and renal salt loss is frequently seen. The polyuria requires large volumes (up to 10 litres/24 h is not uncommon) of intravenous fluid to be given which, given the salt loss, should be predominantly normal saline. Volume replacement with 5% dextrose or dextrose-saline is likely to cause hyponatraemia. This patient is polyuric and intravascularly volume deplete as demonstrated by the postural drop in blood pressure. Water restriction is therefore inappropriate, the correct management being fluid replacement using normal saline, as guided by measurement of the CVP. Twice-normal saline should only be used in life-threatening hyponatraemia of rapid onset. Dialysis would be indicated for significant fluid overload or dangerously high urea or potassium levels, none of which are relevant here. Dialysis is an effective treatment for hyponatraemia but it is inappropriate to expose the patient to the risks of central venous catheter insertion as alternative treatments are available. Dialysis may be problematic as the patient is haemodynamically unstable. There is nothing to support a diagnosis of Addison's disease.

11. E: pH 7.54, $PaCO_2$ 3.2 kPa, PaO_2 8.1 kPa, bicarbonate 24 mmol/l

Typically such a patient will be hypoxaemic and will hyperventilate in an attempt to increase their PaO_2. This 'blowing off' of CO_2 results in a respiratory alkalosis, which may be compensated for in the more chronic state by renal adjustments of bicarbonate level. However, in the acute state as in this scenario, the arterial blood gases will resemble those seen in acute pulmonary embolism or pneumothorax, i.e. respiratory alkalosis with hypoxaemia. With exhaustion, these patients will retain CO_2 as in any respiratory disease with exhaustion.

12. E: Magnetic resonance imaging (MRI) of the cervical spine

The recent limb weakness and the presence of pyramidal signs in the legs in patients with RA are highly suggestive of a spinal cord lesion at the cervical or thoracic region. RA primarily affects the cervical spine. Involvement of the thoracic or lumbar spine is rare. The anatomical abnormalities occur as a consequence of the destruction of synovial joints, ligaments, and bone. Atlanto-axial subluxation (AAS) is the most common. Patients may experience weakness, decreased endurance, gait difficulty, paresthesiaes of the hands, and loss of fine dexterity. Multiple neurological signs may be elicited on physical examination, including diffuse hyper-reflexia, lower extremity spasticity, a spastic gait, and Babinski's sign.

Although plain radiographs of the cervical spine are regarded as the initial imaging assessment tool for neck pain in patients with RA, those with symptoms or signs of cord compression should undergo immediate MRI and be sent for surgical consultation. MRI is considered the most sensitive imaging technique for diagnosing spinal cord compression, evaluating its extent, and assessing soft tissue (pannus) and the extent of bone destruction. There is no clinical evidence of muscle disease or peripheral neuropathy in this patient and so EMG or NCS are not necessary. Isotope bone scan is a sensitive test and will identify increased activity in the cervical region but it is not specific and plays little part in investigating spinal cord compression.

13. D: Liver biopsy would show features of bridging necrosis

Ferritin is an acute phase protein and may be elevated in inflammatory conditions within and outside the liver. With increasing use of laboratory tests, the pattern of presentation at the time of diagnosis of haemochromatosis has changed. About three-quarters of patients with haemochromatosis are identified by abnormalities in the blood tests performed during routine health check-ups or for symptoms unrelated to iron overloading. Over 90% of patients with genetic haemochromatosis would be either homozygous for the C282Y mutation in the *HFE* gene (previously called *HLA-H*) or compound heterozygotes (heterozygous for the C282Y mutation as well as homo/heterozygous for the H63D mutation). Homozygosity for the H63D alone does not lead to iron overload in the absence of C282Y mutation.

Non-alcoholic fatty liver disease (NAFLD) encompasses simple hepatic steatosis (pure fatty liver) as well as steatohepatitis (NASH). The latter on liver biopsy resembles changes seen in alcoholic hepatitis (ballooning degeneration, Mallory bodies, pericellular or portal fibrosis), hence its name. Both NAFLD and NASH are associated with diabetes, obesity and other states of insulin resistance.

Ultrasound appearances are neither sensitive nor specific in detecting inflammation or fibrosis in the liver.

Drug-induced liver disease can occasionally be associated with the presence of autoantibodies, but a very high titre of smooth muscle antibody (SMA) is rare. SMA has been reported in drug-induced hepatotoxicity due to nitrofurantoin and oxyphenisatin. The hepatocelluar pattern of liver injury, raised IgG and positive SMA is characteristic of autoimmune hepatitis (AIH) type 1. Liver biopsy would show periportal inflammation, which extends beyond the limiting plate (piecemeal necrosis), bridging two portal triads or the central vein. The presence and the degree of fibrosis will relate to the extent and duration of inflammation. AIH type 2 would have positive liver-kidney-microsomal (LKM) antibodies and type 3, antibody to soluble liver antigen (SLA). Anti-double-stranded DNA antibody is characteristic of systemic lupus erythematosus.

14. E: Warfarin to an INR of 2–3.5

Patients with atrial fibrillation (AF), whether persistent, intermittent or chronic, should be anticoagulated if they have an embolic event. The carotid bruit in this case should be regarded as a marker of vascular disease rather than the causal lesion because the history is of a left anterior circulation lesion and the bruit is on the right. Nevertheless, Doppler ultrasound of both carotids should be undertaken. Two main mechanisms are thought to trigger vascular events in AF: the widely recognised issue is of clot forming in and embolising from the left atrial appendage; less well recognised is sluggish flow through the atria causing partial activation of the clotting cascade and a generalised thrombotic tendency.

Appropriate therapy in AF is related to baseline thrombosis risk: no anticoagulation is required in young patients with sustained lone AF (with no other vascular disease and structurally normal hearts). However, there is a much higher risk in even intermittent AF with other vascular risks and anticoagulation may be warranted in such patients.

15. D: Metronidazole

Antibiotic-associated colitis is caused by overgrowth of *Clostridium difficile*, which is a normal large bowel commensal. It is usually seen in relation to broad-spectrum antibiotics, which suppress or eradicate other colonic flora and allow *C. difficile* colonisation. Oral metronidazole and oral vancomycin are active against the organism. Note that oral vancomycin is not normally absorbed after oral administration, so its effects are confined to the gastrointestinal tract.

16. D: (–0.83 to –0.77)

The 95% confidence interval is constructed approximately from the mean ± 2 standard errors. The standard error can be calculated by dividing the standard deviation by the square root of the sample size. Hence, in this question, standard error = $0.15/\sqrt{100}$ = 0.15/10 = 0.015; and the 95% confidence interval = $(-0.8 \pm (2 \times 0.015))$ = (-0.8 ± 0.03) = (–0.83 to –0.77).

D is therefore correct.

The least correct is B (only one potential confidence limit is given).

The nearest correct is A where the 95% range (mean ± 2 sd) is given rather than the 95% confidence interval.

There is no basis for choosing C or E although these might look appealing because of the degree of precision.

17. C: Granuloma annulare

All of the listed conditions are associated with diabetes mellitus. Granuloma annulare commonly affects the hands, feet, knees and elbows, and may occur in both localised or generalised forms. Necrobiosis lipoidica starts as an erythematous plaque with a central atrophic yellowish centre, and usually occurs on the lower limbs. Diabetic dermopathy begins with dull papules on the shins which heal with atrophic brown scars. Diabetic bullae appear spontaneously as blisters on the extremities, usually in elderly diabetics. Tinea infection, although annular in pattern, classically presents with a peripheral powdery scale.

18. B: Primary hyperparathyroidism

An incidental finding of a high calcium level, with normal renal function and an inappropriately high PTH, could only be primary hyperparathyroidism. Patients with hypercalcaemia of malignancy are usually ill, and their PTH (if measured) is appropriately suppressed. Secondary and tertiary hyperparathyroidism are most commonly found in the context of renal failure: in secondary hyperparathyroidism, the PTH is elevated in response to hypocalcaemia. This may also be seen in osteomalacia.

19. B: Myelofibrosis

Myelofibrosis is characterised by progressive fibrosis of the bone marrow with the development of haematopoiesis in the liver and spleen. Fibrosis is a secondary phenomenon due to hyperplasia of megakaryocytes. It is typically a disease of older people and presents with an insidious onset with symptoms of anaemia. Hypermetabolic features such as sweating, weight loss, anorexia and gout are common. Laboratory features include anaemia, raised white cell and platelet counts early in the disease but leucopenia and thrombocytopenia at a later stage. A leukoerythroblastic blood picture with 'teardrop' poikilocytes is classic. It is frequently impossible to aspirate bone marrow and 'a dry tap' and fibrosis with increased megakaryocytes is seen on the trephine. Raised serum urate and LDH reflect the increased cell turnover. Treatment is largely palliative, aimed at reducing symptoms.

20. D: Left thalamic metastasis
The dense sensory impairment described here is typical of a space-occupying thalamic lesion, and the progressive history over several months makes metastasis more likely than either demyelination or stroke. Sensory loss caused by a cortical lesion is rarely complete.

21. C: Refsum disease
The features are consistent with Refsum disease, which may present in adult life. This syndrome also includes peripheral neuropathy and ichthyosis.

22. D: Necrotising fasciitis
Crepitus indicates the presence of gas forming organisms within the subcutaneous tissues. Typically, necrotising fasciitis is very tender and has a higher incidence in diabetics. An infected thrombophlebitis, local abscess and superficial cellulitis would not cause crepitus. Urgent surgical exploration and debridement, together with broad-spectrum antibiotic cover, is indicated.

23. A: Burning on micturition
Urinary symptoms can occur in anxiety but usually consist of frequency or urgency. Chest discomfort at rest, often over the heart, can occur in anxiety. Diarrhoea and constipation can both occur in anxiety, as can the complaint of a difficulty in swallowing.

24. B: Amoxicillin and flucloxacillin
The commonest organism in community-acquired pneumonia is still *Streptococcus pneumoniae* and therefore she **must** receive anti-streptococcal antibiotics, e.g. amoxicillin. However, following influenza one must always consider *Staphylococcus aureus* and treat this e.g. with flucloxacillin, but **always** remembering to cover *Streptococcus pneumoniae* as well. The combination of erythromycin and rifampicin is used to treat Legionnaire's disease.

25. B: Episcleritis

Approximately 25% of patients with rheumatoid arthritis (RA) will have ocular manifestations: keratoconjunctivitis sicca, episcleritis, scleritis, keratitis, peripheral corneal ulceration; and other less common conditions such as choroiditis, retinal vasculitis, episcleral nodules, retinal detachments, and macular edema. Keratoconjunctivitis sicca, or dry eye syndrome, is the most common ocular manifestation of RA and has a reported prevalence of 15–25%. However, painless red eyes in patients with RA are most often a manifestation of episcleritis. The prevalence of scleritis and episcleritis in patients with RA is 4–10%. Scleritis and episcleritis are distinguished on the basis of anatomy and appearance. Symptoms may be similar, but the pain in scleritis is more severe. Tenderness to palpation of the globe can help differentiate the two. After asking the patient to look down with eyelids closed, the physician gently presses the globe. Patients with scleritis have tenderness on palpation; those with episcleritis do not. Unlike patients with scleritis, patients with episcleritis do not complain of blurred vision or photophobia. Correctly diagnosing and distinguishing between scleritis and episcleritis is important because of the potential ocular and systemic complications associated with scleritis. Studies have shown that patients with RA-associated scleritis have more widespread systemic disease and a higher mortality rate than those with episcleritis.

26. B: Rheumatic fever

Diagnosis of rheumatic fever requires serological or microbiological evidence of recent group A streptococcal infection and the application of the Duckett Jones criteria. Two major criteria (pancarditis, polyarthritis, chorea, erythema marginatum, subcutaneous nodules) or one major and two minor criteria (arthralgia, fever, raised ESR/CRP/WCC, conduction defect, previous rheumatic fever) are required to make the diagnosis. Coxsackie B virus is a potent cause of carditis and may also cause arthralgia. The systemic form, Still's disease, has a similar presentation but the cardiac features are less pronounced and joint involvement tends to be delayed. Sarcoidosis is protean in its presentation and can almost never be discounted in systemic disease questions but, as with SLE, such a florid cardiac presentation would be very unusual.

27. E: Drug-induced renal sodium loss

Pseudohyponatraemia is seen when plasma sodium is measured by either an indirect-reading ion-selective electrode or flame photometry, both of which measure sodium in total plasma (solid and water phases) – excess 'solid', e.g. lipid or protein, is present in the sample, 'diluting' the plasma sodium, which is present only in the water phase. If measured with a direct-reading ion-selective electrode the true sodium concentration in plasma water is measured and the presence of excess solid does not affect plasma sodium measurement. A minority of analyses are performed using a direct-reading ion-selective electrode. The history here does not suggest the patient has hyperlipidaemia of a magnitude to cause pseudohyponatraemia.

Drug-induced diabetes insipidus is caused by drugs which either decrease ADH secretion (neurogenic) or decrease the response of the kidney to ADH (nephrogenic). Alcohol is the commonest and induces a diuresis by inhibiting ADH release. These drugs would cause hypernatraemia, not hyponatraemia. There is nothing in the history to point to Addison's disease. SIADH is a recognised complication of bronchial neoplasm but can also rarely complicate cerebrovascular accident. Although both are possible in this patient, the history specifically states that he is taking carbamazepine. Carbamazepine is a well-recognised cause of hyponatraemia and indeed may be used to treat diabetes insipidus. The mechanism responsible for this action remains unclear, but effects on both ADH release and renal response to ADH have been demonstrated.

28. B: High first-pass metabolism of orally administered GTN

GTN is subject to extensive hepatic metabolism, and high first-pass metabolism. As a result, oral administration results in very low systemic bioavailability. The sublingual route results in rapid systemic absorption across the mucous membranes, providing prompt relief from ischaemic symptoms. Nitrate tolerance is more likely to occur in the setting of prolonged nitrate exposure and is more commonly encountered during use of transdermal patches: for this reason patches should be removed for at least six hours daily to allow a nitrate-free period.

29. B: Uroporphyrinogen decarboxylase

Uroporphyrinogen decarboxylase is reduced in activity in porphyria cutanea tarda, which is the most common porphyria. The acquired form is often associated with excess alcohol consumption, and is usually managed by sun avoidance, reduced alcohol intake, venesection and chloroquine. A simple bedside test is to screen the urine with Wood's light, which will fluoresce coral pink due to the presence of excess urinary uroporphyrins.

30. E: 24-hour oesophageal pH study is indicated for the diagnosis of gastro-oesophageal reflux disease in those who have no endoscopic abnormalities

Gastro-oesophageal reflux disease (GORD) is a common condition, with about 10% of the population experiencing the symptoms at some point in time. Twenty-four-hour oesophageal pH monitoring is the most useful test for the diagnosis of GORD in those with negative endoscopy. Abnormally low oesophageal pH for a significant period during 24-hour recording would confirm the diagnosis. A symptom diary, with pH monitoring, will assist in correlation of symptoms with acid reflux. Endoscopic examination is useful to demonstrate oesophagitis, which is present in only half of patients suffering from GORD. A further 15% can be identified by histological examination of biopsy from the gastro-oesophageal junction. Although the characteristic findings of an irregular Z-line with red tongues of columnar lining extending into the oesophagus can be identified at endoscopy, biopsy is essential to distinguish between columnar-lined oesophagus with gastric metaplasia and intestinal metaplasia. Barrett's columnar-lined oesophagus with intestinal metaplasia has been considered to progress in a small proportion of subjects to adenocarcinoma of the oesophagus. Radiological demonstration of barium reflux and demonstration of low oesophageal sphincter tone do not distinguish physiological reflux and have poor correlation with symptoms. Proton pump inhibitors are the drugs of choice for gastro-oesophageal reflux, with a healing rate of more than 90% when used in those with oesophagitis.

31. C: Isotope scan of the thyroid

The differential diagnosis includes Graves 'thyrotoxicosis, postpartum thyroiditis, and a toxic multinodular goitre. Thyrotoxicosis due to postpartum thyroiditis is a self-limiting, transient condition. An isotope scan of the thyroid would best enable you to distinguish between the diagnoses. In the thyrotoxic phase of postpartum thyroiditis, the thyroid gland is 'cold' on an isotope scan, as it is 'spitting out' preformed thyroid hormone, rather than synthesising more. Remember that the thyroid autoantibody titre is not always positive in patients with Graves' disease.

32. E: A Rh-positive

AB Rh-positive and -negative and B Rh-positive blood are incompatible in this patient who will have anti-B antibodies. If at all possible group-compatible blood should be used rather than group O. The problem with this lady, who is nulliparous, is that if she is given

A Rh-positive blood she may make an anti-D antibody which could interfere with future reproduction. However, in a life threatening situation it is the best option. If she is given Rh-positive blood and survives then she should be given anti-D to try to stop the formation of an anti-D antibody.

33. A: Haem

Severe, symmetric polyneuropathy, together with abdominal pain and neuropsychiatric symptoms (or confusion), is typical of acute intermittent porphyria. This is a disorder of haem metabolism inherited as an autosomal dominant syndrome, with attacks often precipitated by drugs, such as oestrogens, phenytoin and sulphonamides. The neuropathy often involves the motor nerves more severely than the sensory; symptoms may begin in the arms or legs, usually distally but occasionally also in the proximal limb girdle.

34. E: Anterior ischaemic optic neuropathy

At this age an ischaemic cause is the most likely. Demyelination would be most likely in a young patient.

35. E: Acute hepatitis E

Hepatitis E is a zoonosis transmitted by the faecal–oral route. Drinking water is contaminated in the rainy season. In endemic areas most people will have caught hepatitis A by the age of five, so acute hepatitis A in an adult would be very unusual. The incubation period is too short for acute hepatitis B (two to six months). Although leptospirosis causes jaundice, it only extremely rarely causes a frank hepatitis and hepatic failure. Yellow fever does not occur in Asia.

36. B: Obsessional impulse

Obsessions are defined as recurrent thoughts that keep re-entering an individual's mind, even though the individual tries to exclude them. They are recognised by the individual as their own thought. Types of obsessions include thoughts, ruminations, doubts and impulses. Rituals are associated with compulsions.

37. B: Nephrocalcinosis may occur

The biochemical abnormality is hyperchloraemic acidosis with associated hypokalaemia. The urine pH is inappropriately high given the acidosis, suggesting an inability to acidify the urine. The anion gap is normal. The diagnosis of type 1 (distal) renal tubular acidosis (RTA) is confirmed by the failure to acidify the urine following acid loading. Sjögren's syndrome is a well recognised association with type 1 RTA.

Proximal RTA (type 2) is due to a failure to reabsorb bicarbonate. Distal RTA is due to a failure to excrete acid due to abnormal ammonia genesis. Proximal RTA is associated with Fanconi syndrome and osteomalacia. Type 1 RTA is associated with nephrocalcinosis. Out-of-date tetracycline has been demonstrated to cause tubular damage leading to proximal RTA.

38. A: 180/205

The following table can be constructed:

	Tuberculosis		
	Yes	No	
Test: Positive	180	25	205
Negative	20	295	315
	200	320	520

Sensitivity = 180/200 (answer D is therefore incorrect).
Specificity = 295/320 (answer B is therefore incorrect).
Positive predictive value = 180/205 (answer A is correct).
Negative predictive value = 295/315 (answer E is therefore incorrect but next nearest to correct).
Proportion in agreement = (180+295)/520 = 475/520 (answer C is incorrect and possibly the least correct because this is not a statistic that would generally be applied to screening type studies).

39. D: Interstitial infiltrates

There is a simple staging system for the chest X-ray in sarcoidosis and the higher the stage, the worse is the prognosis: stage 0 = normal chest X-ray; stage 1 = bilateral hilar lymphadenopathy (BHL); stage 2 = BHL + interstitial infiltrates; stage 3 = interstitial infiltrates only; stage 4 = diffuse fibrosis. Therefore, in the presence of interstitial infiltrates it is better to have coexistent BHL.

40. B: Anticardiolipin antibodies

The tendency for abnormal blood clotting at this relatively young age raises the possibility of thrombophilia. The commonest cause of thrombophilia is hereditary resistance to activated protein C. A variant produced by a mutation in the factor V gene, factor V Leiden, leads to slowed inactivation of the factor V molecule by its inhibitor, protein C. Other congenital causes of thrombophilia include antithrombin III deficiency, protein C deficiency and protein S deficiency. None of the above mentioned causes is associated with prolonged APTT. The clinical picture and blood abnormality is consistent with the diagnosis of antiphospholipid syndrome. Clinical manifestations include fetal loss and arterial or venous thrombosis, thrombocytopenia and the presence of antiphospholipid antibodies. The antiphospholipid antibodies may be suggested by the detection of anticardiolipin antibodies or the lupus anticoagulant.

41. A: Endoscopic retrograde cholangiopancreatography (ERCP) would be diagnostic of primary sclerosing cholangitis (PSC)

Minocycline causes a hepatocellular pattern of liver injury associated with positive ANA and anti-DNA antibody. A cholestatic pattern of liver injury in this clinical context is suggestive of PSC. About 5% of patients with ulcerative colitis develop PSC and most would have pancolitis with minimal symptoms. On the other hand, 75% of patients with PSC have ulcerative colitis. Most patients are male, with the onset before the age of 45 years. There is an association with other autoimmune conditions such as Sjögren's syndrome, Riedel's thyroiditis. Up to 87% of patients with PSC have the perinuclear-staining type of anti-neutrophil cytoplasmic antibodies (pANCA). Inflammation of both the intra- and extrahepatic biliary system leads to fibro-obliterative cholangiopathy. ERCP is the investigation of choice and shows characteristic multiple strictures interspersed along the biliary system, giving a beaded appearance, in 95% of patients. The rest of the patients may have what is known as 'small duct PSC' in which liver biopsy demonstrates concentric sleeves of fibrous tissue surrounding injured bile duct epithelium. Cholangiocarcinoma is a complication of PSC occurring in about 10% of all PSC patients and has been found in 30% of the livers at transplantation or autopsy. About one-third of these cases are diagnosed within the first year of diagnosis. Patients with PSC are at higher risk of colorectal carcinoma.

42. D: Implantable defibrillator

In patients with significantly impaired left ventricular (LV) function, syncope is due to ventricular tachycardia (VT) until proved otherwise. NICE recommends screening patients with prior infarcts and ejection fractions below 0.35 with ambulatory ECG and, if non-sustained VT is seen, an electrophysiological study. Patients with inducible VT should then be offered an implantable defibrillator. Many would argue that ischaemic heart disease with LVEF < 0.3 justifies primary prevention of sudden death with a defibrillator without further risk stratification (MADIT II trial). Defibrillators are superior to amiodarone in the treatment and secondary prevention of VT/VF (AVID trial). Bradycardia is possible but less likely. Carotid stenosis might produce transient ischaemic attacks but these seldom cause syncope without other neurological effects.

43. C: Increased aldosterone production

Hydrocortisone is a natural corticosteroid that binds principally to the glucocorticoid receptor and, to a lesser extent, to the mineralocorticoid receptor. Its secretion is stimulated by ACTH; hydrocortisone administration reduces ACTH release through negative feedback mechanisms. Although aldosterone is also synthesised by the adrenal glands, it is under the control of the renin-angiotensin-aldosterone system and not influenced by ACTH. Corticosteroids cause a non-specific impairment of many of the processes involved in inflammation and, consequently, hydrocortisone increases the risk of infection. In addition to salt and water retention, hydrocortisone promotes hypokalaemia and glucose intolerance and increases gastric acid production.

44. C: Sagittal sinus

Parasagittal bi-parietal or bi-frontal hemorrhagic infarctions are common sequelae of sagittal sinus thrombosis. Oral contraceptives, the immediate postpartum period, hypercoagulable states, and dehydration all predispose to sagittal sinus thrombosis. The presence of multiple lesions which are not in typical arterial territories, and the prominent epileptic fits, favour this diagnosis.

45. E: Alopecia areata

Alopecia areata is a form of hair loss suspected to have an immunological basis due to its association with autoimmune disease. The scalp is the first site to be affected in over 60% of cases but bald patches may occur in the beard, eyebrows or eyelashes. Androgenetic alopecia refers to male-pattern baldness, telogen effluvium to diffuse hair loss following an episode of severe illness and folliculitis decalvans to an inflammatory process affecting hair follicles which causes scarring.

46. A: Aldosterone:renin ratio

This could be Conn's syndrome (primary hyperaldosteronism). As a general rule in endocrinology, remember to make the biochemical diagnosis before undertaking any imaging: adrenal 'incidentalomas' are common, (as are pituitary 'incidentalomas'). You should also avoid screening for diagnoses if the clinical suspicion is low, as this increases the risk of false-positive results (e.g. looking for Cushing's syndrome in a patient with no signs of the condition). As the patient has hypertensive retinopathy, you do not need to confirm the diagnosis of poorly controlled hypertension.

47. E: Delayed haemolytic transfusion reaction

This is a typical story of a delayed haemolytic transfusion reaction. The patient was transfused 35 years ago as an emergency following the birth of her second child. She is Kell negative and was exposed to a Kell-positive unit at that time and developed anti-Kell antibody. However she has not had any exposure to blood products since so the antibody was undetectable on screening pre-surgery. She was then transfused with 4 units of blood, 3 of which were Kell-positive. The anti-Kell antibody level rises over the few days following surgery and starts to destroy the Kell-positive transfused cells, causing anaemia and jaundice. Her direct antiglobulin test is now positive and anti-Kell can easily be detected on antibody screening.

48. C: Tuberose sclerosis

Theses lesions are seen most commonly in tuberose sclerosis, but are also associated with neurofibromatosis.

49. D: Haloperidol

All antipsychotics can reduce the seizure threshold and so should be used with caution in epilepsy. Clozapine and zotepine in particular affect the seizure threshold adversely. There is limited data on the newer antipsychotics, so for individuals whose epilepsy is not well controlled, it may be safer to use more established antipsychotics. From this group, haloperidol is preferable to chlorpromazine. Doxepin is an antidepressant.

50. E: Coxsackievirus

The story is most compatible with an acute viral myocarditis and pulmonary oedema. Wheeze and an elevated venous pressure are not usually features of SARS, *Mycoplasma* and Q fever (although Q fever is acquired from sheep), but respiratory infections like *Mycoplasma* can rarely cause a myocarditis too. It is very unusual (but not impossible) to have such a prolonged fall in CD4 count during acute HIV seroconversion that *Pneumocystis carinii* pneumonia can develop.

51. C: pH 7.38, PaCO$_2$ 5.3 kPa, PaO$_2$ 8.1 kPa, bicarbonate 30 mmol/l

This man has features of life-threatening asthma (PEFR < 33%, feeble respiratory effort). This type of case should be managed in the ICU/HDU setting as he is at a higher risk of death. This type of case may require prophylactic intubation and ventilation to prevent respiratory arrest while waiting for bronchodilators and corticosteroids to take effect. With respect to the arterial blood gases, if the $PaCO_2$ is normal/high an anaesthetic colleague should be called urgently as the patient is tiring and may have a respiratory arrest. The $PaCO_2$ should be low in an acute attack because of hyperventilation.

52. D: Salicylate overdose

In metabolic acidosis the bicarbonate will be low, requiring an increase in anions in order to maintain electrochemical balance. It is important to remember that any acid is composed of hydrogen ions and an equivalent amount of anions. If the metabolic acidosis is due to an excess of either endogenous or exogenous acid (e.g. diabetic ketoacidosis, lactic acidosis, salicylate poisoning), the hydrogen ions are associated with an equivalent amount of unmeasured anions. Therefore, no compensatory increase in chloride is necessary as the anions carry a negative charge, electrochemical balance remaining undisturbed. The anion gap (unmeasured anions) will be increased and the chloride normal. If the metabolic acidosis is not due to excess acid plus anions (e.g. bicarbonate loss in proximal renal tubular acidosis) the anion gap will be normal and a compensatory rise in chloride will be seen. This patient is acidotic with a calculated anion gap of 20 mmol/l and normal chloride. Thus the source of exogenous anions or excessive endogenous anion generation should be sought. Endogenous anions may be ketoacids as seen in diabetic ketoacidosis, or the numerous unmeasured anions that accumulate in renal failure. The normal blood glucose and creatinine exclude these. Exogenous anions include lactate (lactic acidosis) and, as in this case, salicylate. Paracetamol and triclyclic antidepressants do not cause acid–base disturbance directly.

53. A: Antinuclear antibody (ANA)

Almost all patients with SLE have positive ANA test results. The ANA test is sensitive but not specific for SLE. A negative result argues strongly against a diagnosis of active SLE, but does not exclude the possibility of other autoimmune diseases.

Antibodies to Sm antigen are highly specific for a diagnosis of SLE (> 99%). However, only about 25% of patients with SLE have anti-Sm antibodies. Anti-dsDNA antibodies are diagnostic of SLE (specificity > 99%). However, only 60% of patients with SLE will have these antibodies. Therefore, absence of anti-dsDNA or anti-Sm antibodies should not exclude SLE as a diagnosis. Anti-Ro (SSA) antibodies are found in 30% of patients with SLE. Antihistone antibodies are identified in small proportion of SLE patients. They are more often seen with drug-induced lupus.

54. D: Immune-mediated thrombocytopenia

Abciximab is a monoclonal antibody to the glycoprotein IIb/IIIa receptor. It binds and inhibits this receptor, which is the final common pathway of platelet activation. Being immunologically active it potentiates autoimmune platelet destruction. DIC and marrow toxicity are not recognised effects. Myelofibrosis can cause very low platelet counts but one would expect to have picked this up before the procedure. Tirofiban is an alternative IIb/IIIa inhibitor licensed in acute coronary syndromes; it is not a monoclonal antibody.

55. E: Dose of drug

V_d is the apparent volume of distribution of drug, and is a theoretical volume based on the administered dose (D) and plasma concentration (C) ($V_d = D/C$). It does not necessarily conform to physiological volumes and widely distributed drugs, e.g. amiodarone, can have a V_d that is considerably greater than total body water volume. Drugs with a low V_d (e.g. 4 l) are predominantly confined to the plasma space, and likely to be water soluble, highly protein-bound with low tissue binding. Drugs with a high V_d tend to be lipid soluble, with a low degree of protein binding and high tissue binding. The ratio of body fat to lean muscle is likely to influence lipophilic drugs that tend to be widely distributed in peripheral tissues. Serum albumin concentrations influence the extent of protein binding and, therefore, the volume of distribution. V_d is thought to remain constant across a range of doses, such that the plasma drug concentration is proportional to dose (C = D/ V_d).

56. B: Genetic testing for FAP can be performed using DNA from white blood cells obtained by venepuncture

FAP is inherited as an autosomal dominant disorder which occurs in about 1 in 10,000 births. FAP and Gardner's syndrome arise from mutations of the adenomatous polyposis coli (APC) gene on chromosome 5, which is a tumour suppressor gene. The condition is characterised by hundreds to thousands of colonic adenomas, which develop at an average age of 16 years. Polyps are usually distributed uniformly throughout the colon. Virtually all affected individuals develop polyposis by the age of 35 years and the average age for developing colonic cancer is 39 years. Extra-colonic manifestations include desmoid tumours, osteomas, CHRPE, supernumerary teeth and soft tissue skin tumours. The term 'Gardner's syndrome' is used when extra-intestinal features are predominant. Genetic testing should be done for FAP after the age of 12 years to avoid adverse effects on the self-image and concerns over peer rejection. Genetic testing can be done using white blood cell DNA purified from venous blood, which would identify mutations in virtually 100% of the family members. Subtotal colectomy has been advocated by some to prevent the development of colorectal cancer in susceptible individuals.

Peutz-Jeghers syndrome is inherited as an autosomal dominant condition characterised by hamartomatous gastrointestinal polyps and cutaneous pigmentation around the lips and nose. Juvenile polyps are hamartomas, which occur most commonly in the colon. About one-third of these individuals have an inherited form and the rest are sporadic cases.

HNPCC is an autosomal dominant condition characterised by the occurrence of colorectal cancer around the age of 45 years. The 'Amsterdam' criteria for diagnosis of this disease are:

1. Three family members with colon cancer
2. The cases spanning at least two generations
3. At least one of the cases diagnosed under the age of 50 years.

Seventy percent of the tumours in HNPCC occur in the proximal colon. HNPCC is caused by mutations of any of the four DNA mismatch repair genes which repair errors introduced by DNA polymerase during cell replication.

57. C: Subungal fibromas

The girl has tuberose sclerosis which is inherited as an autosomal dominant condition. There is some genetic heterogeneity but abnormalities have been linked with chromosomes 9 and 11. It is characterised by epilepsy, mental retardation, retinal phakomas, ash-leaf macules, adenoma sebaceum, peri- and subungual fibromas, shagreen patches, and renal and cardiac hamartomas.

58. A: Vitamin B_{12} deficiency

Subacute combined degeneration of the spinal cord, caused by vitamin B_{12} deficiency, results in degeneration of the posterior columns (vibration and joint-position sense), followed by progressive development of upper motor neurone signs in the legs. Spinal cord involvement is roughly symmetrical, but can progress to dementia and visual impairment due to optic neuropathy. Thiamine deficiency may give rise to Wernicke's syndrome (ophthalmoplegia, ataxia and confusion) or to beri-beri (peripheral neuropathy). Pyridoxine deficiency gives rise to a chronic painful sensorimotor neuropathy. This can be caused by administration of isoniazid (for tuberculosis), which increases the excretion of pyridoxine; isoniazid is therefore always administered in conjunction with pyridoxine.

59. D: Maturity-onset diabetes of the young (MODY)

Prompts to think about MODY include the patient's young age, slim build (making an early presentation of type 2 diabetes less likely), lack of ketonuria, and his unusual family history (of early-onset, diet-controlled diabetes). However, MODY is rare, and atypical presentations of type 1 or type 2 diabetes should always be considered. In particular, patients with Type 1 diabetes may not have ketonuria at presentation: any decision to treat a young, newly diagnosed diabetic with diet or tablets should be extremely carefully monitored.

60. A: Iron deficiency anaemia

These indices are typical of severe iron deficiency anaemia with a pronounced hypochromic microcytic anaemia and decreased red cell count. The platelet count is frequently raised reactively as the marrow attempts to compensate. Iron deficiency is caused by inadequate intake of iron (dietary, pregnancy, growth spurts), malabsorption, (coeliac disease, gastrectomy) or blood loss (from the gastrointestinal tract, uterus, urinary tract or lungs). This case was due to a very poor diet. Management consists of oral iron, starting with the cheapest preparation, oral ferrous sulphate. With good compliance one would expect a rapid response in a case like this.

61. E: Serological testing for herpes simplex virus (HSV) IgG

A positive or negative result to this test is not going to allow any therapeutic decision to be made, or health advice to be given, apart from warning him that he may contract primary HSV if the test is negative. HSV is treated on the basis of symptoms rather than serology. All of the other tests could lead to possible therapeutic interventions.

62. D: Myasthenia gravis

Failure of upgaze alone, with preservation of other eye movements, excludes a third cranial nerve palsy. Ptosis does not occur in dysthyroid eye disease and eye movements would be normal in Horner's syndrome.

63. D: Thought echo

Thought echo is the experience of hearing one's thoughts repeated out loud and is a first-rank symptom of schizophrenia. First-rank symptoms, in the absence of organic disease, are strongly suggestive of schizophrenia. Other first-rank symptoms include third-person auditory hallucinations, running-commentary hallucinations, somatic hallucinations, delusional perceptions, thought alienation and made feelings or actions believed to be due to the influence of others (passivity).

64. C: Splenomegaly

Bad prognostic indicators for sarcoidosis include: age > 40 years, stage 3 disease, symptoms for > 6 months, more than three organs involved, absence of erythema nodosum, splenomegaly. The spleen may become very enlarged and require careful surgical removal to prevent haemorrhage.

65. A: Further stone formation may be prevented by D-penicillamine treatment

The history is of ureteric obstruction. The ground-glass appearance of the calculi is diagnostic of cystine stones. The essence of management of any urinary calculi is maintenance of an adequate urinary volume and minimisation of solute excretion. Increased fluid intake is therefore important in cystinuria. D-penicillamine prevents cystine excretion. Cystinuria is associated with increased excretion of other dibasic amino acids (lysine and arginine), but not neutral amino acids, which is seen in Hartnup's disease. Bendroflumethiazide (bendrofluazide) decreases urinary calcium excretion, although urinary oxalate excretion is a more important determinant of calcium oxalate stone formation.

66. C: Psoriatic arthritis

Arthritis with predominant involvement of the distal interphalangeal (DIP) joint occurs most often in generalised osteoarthritis and psoriatic arthritis. The fact that she is relatively young and has a raised ESR indicates that an underlying inflammatory disease is the most likely cause of her symptoms. Psoriatic arthritis is therefore the most likely diagnosis in this case. Rheumatoid arthritis and SLE are known to affect the proximal interphalangeal (PIP) and the metacarpophalangeal (MCP) joints. Chronic gouty arthritis might involve the DIPs, but more often it involves the MCPs and PIPs in an asymmetrical fashion, with or without tophus formation. Examination of the skin and nails for psoriasis is very important in confirming the diagnosis. The hair margin of the scalp, the navel and the palms are areas often involved in psoriasis but easily missed.

67. C: Atrioventricular re-entry tachycardia

Wolff-Parkinson-White (WPW) syndrome is caused by the presence of an accessory pathway between the atria and ventricles. The fast-conducting slow-recovering AV node and slow-conducting fast-recovering accessory pathway fulfill the requirements for a re-entry tachycardia. As this involves both atria and ventricles it is an atrio-ventricular re-entry mechanism. As the QRS duration is shorter in tachycardia than at rest an orthodromic circuit (anterograde through the AV node, retrograde through the accessory pathway) must be operating. In a macro re-entry atrial tachycardia the circuit is limited to the atria and conducted through the AV node, usually with some degree of block. Atrial flutter is the commonest example of this mechanism. Atrial fibrillation is of note in WPW because of the risk of the fibrillation waves bypassing the normal rate-limiting step of the AV node and conducting anterograde down the accessory pathway, degenerating into ventricular fibrillation. Ventricular re-entry indicates a circuit not involving the atria; AV node re-entry indicates a circuit confined to the AV node and its pathways.

68. E: Weight gain

Lithium has a narrow therapeutic range and therapeutic drug monitoring is used to reduce the risk of toxicity. The normal therapeutic range is 0.4–1.0 mmol/l. Serious adverse effects occur above 1.5 mmol/l and are particularly common at concentrations of 2.0 mmol/l or more. Adverse effects include gastrointestinal symptoms (nausea, vomiting and diarrhoea) and neurological symptoms (blurred vision, reduced conscious level, ataxia, tremor, dysarthria). Severe overdosage can result in convulsions, circulatory collapse, hypokalaemia, coma and death. Hypothyroidism occurs more commonly as an adverse effect of chronic administration, but has been reported following acute intoxication. Weight gain is a feature of chronic administration, but not of acute lithium poisoning.

69. D: Ursodeoxycholic acid (UDCA) therapy could delay the need for liver transplantation

Primary biliary cirrhosis (PBC) is a chronic cholestatic liver disease characterised by progressive destruction and disappearance of small intrahepatic bile ducts. The majority of cases of PBC are now identified in the asymptomatic phase, and 90% are women. There is an association between PBC and other autoimmune diseases such as rheumatoid arthritis and Sjögren's syndrome. The serological pattern is most helpful in clinching the diagnosis and antimitochondrial antibody (AMA) is detected in 95% of subjects. There is a polyclonal increase in immunoglobulin levels with a high IgM in particular, as well as IgG in AMA-positive cases. The major antimitochondrial antibody found in PBC patients is called anti-M2 antibody, although the relationship between these and the bile duct injury is not clear. Histologically, there is mononuclear cell damage to the biliary epithelium, classically with non-necrotising epithelioid granuloma formation in the portal triad, progressing through portal fibrosis and eventually to cirrhosis. Specific immunosuppressive therapy with steroids and azathioprine has not been shown to be effective in the long-term management of PBC. Age, ascites, haemoglobin, bilirubin, albumin and prothrombin time are the factors predicting the survival, not the degree of raised liver enzymes. UDCA is a hydrophilic bile acid, which has been shown to reduce itching in some patients. It is well tolerated but causes diarrhoea in about 2% of subjects. UDCA lowers serum bilirubin and significantly prolongs the time before liver transplantation is required. PBC recurs after liver transplantation.

70. C: Contraception
Isotretinoin is a retinoid used to treat acne vulgaris. It is teratogenic and therefore patients must be counselled on the need for effective birth control one month before commencing treatment and for one month after treatment ends. It is associated with dry skin, eye irritation, muscle aches, mood changes and depression, increased uric acid levels, liver abnormalities and hyperlipidaemia. Skeletal hyperostosis is associated with long-term retinoid use only.

71. E: Venous blood sample
In a non-diabetic patient presenting with spontaneous hypoglycaemia, a venous blood sample should be taken before treatment, if at all possible. This is the ideal time to make/exclude several important (though rare) diagnoses, including hypocortisolism or an insulinoma. This may avert the need for a hypoglycaemic stress test or prolonged fast at a later date. Other causes of hypoglycaemia should not be forgotten, including hepatic dysfunction, drugs and alcohol, tumours and 'factitious hypoglycaemia' (due to the inappropriate use of insulin or oral hypoglycaemic agents). Baseline tests should include cortisol, insulin and liver function tests. C-peptide (the other product of the cleavage of pro-insulin, secreted in equimolar concentrations with insulin) may be useful to differentiate an insulinoma from insulin 'abuse'.

72. C: Left parietal lobe
Defects in the visual field help to localise neurological lesions. Visual field defects restricted to one eye are likely to be in the retina or optic nerve. Bi-temporal field defects indicate a lesion in the optic chiasm. Homonymous field defects indicate that the pathology lies posterior to the chiasm. Quadrantanopia most often indicates a lesion either in the optic radiations or the occipital cortex. A superior quadrantanopia indicates a lesion in the temporal optic radiations or the inferior bank of the calcarine (primary visual) cortex. Parietal or superior calcarine lesions will cause an inferior quadrantanopia. Binocular altitudinal hemianopia indicates a bilateral occipital lesion. Such a visual field

defect may occur after embolisation to the top of the basilar artery, infarcting both occipital lobes.

73. D: Carbimazole

The lower limit of the neutrophil count is $2.5 \times 10^9/l$ except in Africans and those from the Middle East, where $1.5 \times 10^9/l$ is acceptable. Recurrent infections are likely to occur when the neutrophil count falls below $0.5 \times 10^9/l$. Selective neutropenia due to individual susceptibility to an agent may follow administration of a large number of different drugs. The mechanism of the neutropenia may be direct toxic damage to a bone marrow precursor cell or the stimulation of an immune mechanism which damages neutrophils or their precursors. A drug-hapten mechanism may be responsible in some cases. Drugs which can induce neutropenia include antibacterials, anticonvulsants, anti-inflammatory drugs, anti-thyroids, hypoglycaemics, phenothiazines, psychotropics, antidepressants and other agents like gold and penicillamine. Carbimazole is associated with neutropenia and patients on this drug must be warned to report symptoms and signs suggestive of infection, especially sore throat. A white cell count should be performed if there is any suggestion of infection.

74. D: Experiencing cravings to have a drink

Although continuing excessive consumption of alcohol from an early age is associated with alcohol dependence, only cravings are part of the alcohol dependence syndrome, as first described by Edwards and Gross (1976). The other six features are withdrawal symptoms, relief drinking to avoid withdrawal symptoms, stereotyped pattern of consumption, the development of tolerance, prominence of drink-seeking behaviour over other activities, and reinstatement of previous pattern of dependency after abstinence.

Edwards G. and Gross M. (1976) Alcohol dependence: provisional description of a clinical syndrome. *British Medical Journal*, 1, 1058

75. A: DNA-gyrase mutation

The usual means of resistance to fluoroquinolones is by a mutation in the *gyrA* gene which encodes a DNA gyrase, the target of fluoroquinolones. Some resistance of Gram-negative organisms to ciprofloxacin may be due to the presence of an efflux membrane transporter, but this doses not appear to be the major mechanism. Ciprofloxacin is not a β-lactamase. Intermediate-level resistance to vancomycin in *Staphylococcus aureus* is achieved by an increase in the bacterial cell wall thickness, reducing permeability. Ribosomes are the target of aminoglycosides, macrolides and tetracyclines.

76. A: Churg-Strauss syndrome

Pleural fluid eosinophilia >10% usually means blood or air in the pleural space. Other causes of pleural fluid eosinophilia include: parapneumonic effusion; malignancy; TB; drug-induced (e.g. bromocriptine, dantrolene, nitrofurantoin); asbestos; paragonimiasis; and Churg-Strauss syndrome. The latter two diagnoses are the only ones that cause eosinophilic effusions with decreased pH and decreased glucose level.

77. D: Microcytosis

The ESR test, which is almost 80 years old, has been used as a general screen for organic disease for many years. It depends on two factors:

1. The number, size and shape of red blood cells
2. The concentration of certain plasma proteins.

The relative contribution of plasma proteins to the ESR at constant red blood cell concentration is as follows: fibrinogen/α_2-globulins/gamma globulins/albumin = 10/5/2/1.

ESR is therefore largely a measure of fibrinogen, which is, of course, an acute phase protein. In chronic inflammation, however, increased quantities of immunoglobulins are present in the bloodstream and these also produce an elevated ESR, although this elevation is not due to an acute phase disturbance. Consequently, a high ESR may not necessarily reflect acute inflammation and this is the explanation, of course, for high ESRs in paraproteinaemias and other conditions where high levels of circulating immunoglobins are encountered. Any disease that changes the shape and size of red blood cells decreases the ESR. Distorted cells, as found in microcytosis and sickle cell disease, do not stack and consequently do not settle far. Diseases that cause the body to make less protein or extra red blood cells also decrease the ESR. On the other hand, anaemia, old age, female gender and pregnancy are associated with increased ESR levels.

78. D: The genetic defect responsible for this condition is located on the short arm of chromosome 16

Renal cysts may be demonstrated in many diseases, the commonest of which is autosomal-dominant polycystic kidney disease (ADPKD). Simple renal cysts are acquired with age. Age-related criteria for the ultrasound diagnosis of ADPKD have been defined: for patients with PKD-1 mutations, two cysts are sufficient for the diagnosis up to 30 years; from 30–59 years, two cysts in each kidney are required; and aged 60 years and above, four cysts in each kidney are required.

Patients with marked renal impairment acquire renal cysts. However, the kidneys are small and echogenic and do not present a diagnostic problem. Onset of disease is very variable and not predicted by onset in parents or siblings. From the start of cyst formation there is then progressive loss of excretory renal function over approximately ten years. Patients presenting late may therefore not reach end-stage renal failure. Cases without a family history may be due either to new mutations or to late onset in the affected parent. Inheritance is autosomal dominant with almost complete penetrance but variable expressivity. Abnormalities in two genes account for almost all cases of ADPKD; *PKD-1* or *PKD-2*. *PKD-1* is located on the short arm of chromosome 16 (16p13) and *PKD-2* on chromosome 4q21. The *PKD-1* mutations account for 85–90% of cases. Patients with *PKD-2* mutations have slightly later onset of disease but are otherwise indistinguishable from patients with *PKD-1* mutations.

79. E: Ventricular tachyarrhythmias

A minority of patients with hypertrophic cardiomyopathy have significant outflow-tract obstruction. With or without this they are still at risk of ventricular arrhythmias which are the commonest mode of death attributable to the condition. Risk stratification should be carried out, high-risk features being: history of syncope, family history of sudden death, and non-sustained VT on Holter monitoring or exercise testing. Consideration should be given to defibrillator implantation in individuals identified as high-risk.

80. A: Request stool sample to be screened for *E. coli* O157:H7

This patient has presented with bloody diarrhoea, with a history of contact, thrombocytopenia, evidence of microangiopathic haemolytic anaemia, and renal failure. The most likely diagnosis in this patient is haemolytic uraemic syndrome (HUS). *E. coli* strain O157:H7 is the commonest cause of post-diarrhoeal HUS, accounting for 85% of such cases, although other organisms such as *Campylobacter* and *Shigella* have also been implicated. *Clostridium welchii* septicaemia is associated with striking haemolysis associated with spherocytosis due to phospholipase, but the most common source of infection is the genitourinary tract.

Most cases of *E. coli* O157:H7 have been linked to ground beef. Incubation period ranges from one to eight days. Illness begins with severe abdominal cramps and non-bloody diarrhoea, which becomes bloody by the second or third day. About one-third of patients have vomiting and two-thirds have abdominal tenderness. The lack of fever, with abdominal pain and tenderness, can lead clinician to suspect non-infectious causes, such as inflammatory bowel disease, ischaemic colitis or intussusception (in children). About 6% of patients develop HUS, which is diagnosed 2–14 days. Young children and the elderly are at the greatest risk of developing HUS. *E. coli* O157:H7 produces toxins called shiga-like toxins because they are homologous to the toxin produced by *Shigella dysenteriae*. The toxins are responsible for HUS. As most clinical laboratories do not routinely screen for this pathogen, specific culture and assay for antigens should be requested.

Although *E. coli* O157:H7 is susceptible to antimicrobials used for enteric infections, treatment does not alter the course of infection or complications. Studies suggest that HUS is more likely to develop in those receiving antibiotic therapy, presumably due to release of toxins.

81. E: The rate of elimination does not increase in response to increased drug doses due to saturation of metabolising enzymes

The majority of drugs observe first-order elimination kinetics: the rate of drug metabolism increases in proportion to the administered dosage (linear relationship), which ensures that overall drug clearance remains constant. Other drugs, e.g. phenytoin, observe zero-order elimination kinetics: the rate of metabolism remains constant despite increases in drug dosage, due to saturation of a metabolic pathway. The consequence is that overall drug clearance falls with increased drug dosage. The clinical significance is that small increases in drug dosage result in significantly greater increases in plasma concentration (non-linear pattern).

82. B: Erythema chronicum migrans

The patient is suffering from Lyme disease which is caused by the spirochaete *Borrelia burgdorferi*, and is transmitted by hard-bodied ticks. Erythema chronicum migrans is the characteristic skin eruption, starting at the site of the tick bite as an erythematous macule and expanding in an annular manner with central clearing. Cardiac and neurological signs develop later. Erythema multiforme and erythema annulare centrifugum are not associated with heart block or cranial nerve palsies; erythema gyratum repens is associated with internal malignancy; erythema ab igne presents with reticulate pigmented erythema due to long-term exposure to local heat.

83. B: Metformin

Metformin was the only oral hypoglycaemic agent shown to have beneficial effects on coronary heart disease in patients with type 2 diabetes in the UK Prospective Diabetes Study. It is also the only one of the choices that will not cause this overweight patient to gain more weight: she may even lose some weight, as it can cause mild anorexia. The patient has no obvious contraindications to metformin therapy (such as renal impairment, hepatic dysfunction or cardiac failure).

84. B: Left abducens nerve

The effects of oculomotor paresis on diplopia can be predicted easily by three rules:

1. The direction in which the distance between the images is at a maximum is the direction of action of the paretic muscles.
2. Paresis of the horizontally acting muscles tends to produce mainly horizontal diplopia.
3. The image projected further from the centre belongs to the paretic eye.

Application of these rules to this clinical scenario suggests that the left sixth cranial nerve is dysfunctional.

85. E: Acute promyelocytic leukaemia

Acute myeloid leukaemia (AML) is defined as 20% or more myeloid blasts in the bone marrow (WHO classification). It is the common form of acute leukaemia in adults and is subdivided on the basis of morphology, immunophenotype and cytogenetics. Acute promyelocytic leukaemia (M3) is characterized by the presence of promyelocytes and the cytogenetic translocation t (15; 17). The promyelocytes have a typical heavily granulated appearance and tend to precipitate disseminated intravascular coagulation, often after starting chemotherapy. If the patient can be supported through the initial haemorrhagic phase the prognosis for this type of AML is good.

86. D: Heroin

Amphetamines, cocaine and phencyclidine (PCP) can all produce acute psychosis. Cannabis is associated with the development of psychotic episodes, particularly in vulnerable individuals. Opiates do not produce psychotic symptoms in individuals with clear consciousness.

87. E: 50%

This question relies on your knowledge of (i) the difference between various oxygen entrainment devices and (ii) basic respiratory physiology. As the man's respiratory rate is normal, he should have a normal level of **alveolar ventilation**: [tidal volume – dead space] × respiratory rate = ([500 ml–150 ml] × 15 breaths/min) = 5250 ml/min. Therefore, with this type of face mask, he will be inhaling 2l/min of oxygen and 3.25l/min of room air (21% O_2). Hence, $FIO_2 = (2 + [0.21 \times 3.25]) / 5.25 = 51\%$. This sort of mask is not recommended when accurate FIO_2 is required (e.g. chronic obstructive pulmonary disease), when a high-flow (venturi) mask is safest. With nasal cannulae the actual FIO_2 delivered will vary with the patient's ventilation.

88. B: Rheumatoid nodule

The long duration (>1 h) of early morning and rest stiffness are highly suggestive of an underlying inflammatory condition. The pelvic radiograph confirms the presence of sacroiliits. Bilateral sacroiliitis is typical in ankylosing spondylitis. The incidence of asymmetric sacroiliitis may be higher in other spodyloarthropathies, e.g. reactive arthritis, Reiter's syndrome, spondylitis associated with psoriasis, or inflammatory bowel disease.

Reiter's syndrome characterised by a triad of arthritis, urethritis, and conjunctivitis. Reiter's syndrome develops in the setting of post-dysenteric or post-venereal illness. The characteristic rashes of keratoderma blennorrhagicum and circinate balanitis may be present. Psoriatic spondyloarthropathy is characterised by psoriatic plaques. The skin involvement may be subtle and should be searched for carefully. The cleft of the buttock, hairline, and penis are not unusually involved. Psoriatic nail changes include onycholysis, yellow nails and nail pitting. Inflammatory bowel disease comprises ulcerative colitis and Crohn's disease. A diagnosis of ankylosing spondylitis may be made when specific features of Reiter's syndrome, psoriasis, or inflammatory bowel disease are absent. Sacroiliitis is also encountered in tuberculosis, sarcoidosis and brucellosis. Rheumatoid arthritis (RA) is not associated with lumbar or sacroiliac joint disease. However, cervical spondylitis and atlanto-axial subluxation are not uncommon features of RA.

89. E: Dengue fever

Dengue fever is endemic and epidemic over much of the tropics and causes huge outbreaks and morbidity. Although a single blood film cannot exclude malaria, the postural drop in blood pressure and petechiae are more typical of dengue fever than malaria (which will also cause a thrombocytopenia). It is rare to see a severe thrombocytopenia in typhoid. Murine typhus (*Rickettsia typhi*) can, however, present a similar picture (although petechiae occur in < 10%), but is much less commonly imported to the UK.

90. C: Ostium secundum atrial septal defect

The auscultation findings of atrial septal defect are related to the increased flow through the right heart. This prevents the normal shortening of right ventricular ejection, which occurs as pulmonary vascular resistance increases in inspiration, and fixes the gap between aortic and pulmonary closure. It also generates a flow murmur across the pulmonary valve. Uncorrected pulmonary hypertension may develop.

Secundum defects are associated with right axis deviation, primum defects with left axis deviation. Primum defects are usually associated with mitral regurgitation and present in childhood. Patent foramen ovale, by definition, produces no haemodynamic effects. Ventricular septal defects generate pansystolic murmurs.

91. C: Erythromycin

Erythromycin is an important hepatic enzyme inhibitor, which can reduce the extent of theophylline metabolism and, therefore, increase serum concentrations. Allopurinol, ciprofloxacin and isoniazid are other hepatic enzyme inhibitors that can also promote theophylline toxicity. Hepatic enzyme inhibitors also reduce the clearance of warfarin, and increase prothrombin time and bleeding risk.

92. D: TGF-β

The commonest cause of renal transplant failure after one year is death of the patient with the graft still functioning. The next commonest is chronic allograft nephropathy. This is characterised by a progressive slow deterioration in graft function associated with proteinuria (rarely nephrotic range) and hypertension. The predominant lesion on renal biopsy is interstitial fibrosis with characteristic vascular changes. There is associated tubular loss and, in some cases, glomerular changes: transplant glomerulopathy. As in other chronic renal diseases where interstitial fibrosis is seen, there is dominant TGF-β detectable. Interferon-γ is produced by activated helper and cytotoxic T cells of the type 1 phenotype and is implicated in acute cellular rejection. TNF-α is produced by activated macrophages and is also implicated in acute cellular rejection. Interleukin-4 is produced by helper T cells of the type 2 phenotype and is essential for antibody responses. It inhibits type 1 immune responses. Interleukin-8 is a chemokine responsible for eosinophil chemotaxis.

93. A: Pityriasis versicolor

Pityriasis versicolor is caused by the fungus *Malassezia furfur*, and presents with reddish/brown macules with a typical fine branny scale. On tanned or pigmented skin, the macules may be hypopigmented. Pityriasis rosea is characterised by a herald patch followed by salmon-pink plaques in a 'Christmas tree' distribution; guttate psoriasis presents with numerous erythematous plaques with scale, but it does not respond to selenium sulphide; cutaneous larva migrans presents with the migration of larvae under the skin, associated with urticarial weals; scabies is caused by the mite *Sarcoptes scabiei* and is extremely itchy.

94. A: Osteomalacia

This patient's osteomalacia may result from dietary deficiencies and little exposure to sunlight. Remember that the calcium may only be 'borderline low', and the alkaline phosphatase only 'borderline high'. The proximal myopathy is characteristic. Primary hypoparathyroidism does not cause an elevated alkaline phosphatase.

95. C: Diclofenac should be withdrawn immediately

Twenty-fold elevation of ALT indicates a hepatocellular pattern of liver injury. When there is more than a ten-fold elevation of ALT, differential diagnoses include acute viral hepatitis, drug-induced hepatotoxicity and ischaemic hepatitis (shock liver). Alcoholic hepatitis does not cause such elevation of ALT. In a subject who is on several potentially hepatotoxic drugs, the temporal relationship between starting each drug and the reaction should be considered. Diclofenac causes idiosyncratic hepatotoxicity with a hepatocellular pattern of liver injury: the majority of the reactions present within the first year of starting the medication and 25% of these occur within the first three months. Positive ANA has been reported in patients with diclofenac-hepatotoxicity and both metabolic and immunological mechanisms may be involved. Prompt recognition and immediate withdrawal is the most important step in the management of these cases as severe drug-induced hepatotoxocity leads to acute hepatic failure in 10% of cases. Factors indicating poor prognosis are age over 40 years, prolonged prothrombin time (>50 s), bilirubin > 300 μmol/L, and the development of encephalopathy (especially more than seven days after the onset of jaundice). Steroid therapy has not been shown to alter the course of drug-induced hepatotoxicity.

96. B: Myelodysplastic syndrome

This patient has a macrocytic anaemia with neutropenia and thrombocytopenia. This is most likely to be myelodysplastic syndrome, the subtype of which will be determined on bone marrow examination. Vitamin B_{12} deficiency and folic acid deficiency cause macrocytic anaemia but the macrocytosis and anaemia are likely to be much more severe than this before they cause neutropenia and thrombocytopenia. Myelodysplastic syndromes are acquired neoplastic disorders of multipotent haemopoietic stem cells. They are characterised by ineffective haematopoiesis leading to cytopenias which cause many of the complications. These disorders may progress to acute leukaemia.

97. D: Central retinal vein occlusion
The unilaterality of this pathology makes a central retinal vein occlusion the most likely cause.

98. B: Derealisation
Derealisation is the unpleasant experience that one's surroundings have lost their sense of reality and depth. It may occur in anxiety, fatigue, temporal lobe epilepsy and psychotic illnesses. Depersonalisation describes the distressing feeling that the person no longer feels real, with a diminished ability to feel and experience emotions and events.

99. E: Benign intracranial hypertension
Benign intracranial hypertension (BIH) is a relatively rare neurological disorder, but more common in obese young women. BIH may present with headache, nausea and vomiting, diplopia, transient visual obscurations, or frank visual loss. BIH results in visual field loss and decreased visual acuity and, untreated, may result in complete blindness. Diagnosis is confirmed by documentation of elevated intracranial pressure, normal neurological findings (except for papilloedema and oculomotor palsies, if present), absence of a space-occupying lesion or ventricular enlargement, and normal cerebrospinal fluid. Drug-induced BIH has been reported with tetracyclines, oral contraceptives, nalidixic acid, corticosteroids, nitrofurantoin and etretinate.

100. C: Pulmonary vascular disease
First of all decide if there is a problem to start with, i.e. if the patient reaches 80% of their VO_2max then there is not a significant problem. This man's VO_2max is < 80% predicted so there is a problem but is it pulmonary or circulatory? A normal subject should reach 80% of target heart rate (220 − age in years) but **NOT** reach 80% of their predicted VEmax. This patient only reaches 51% of his maximum ventilation, which tells us that the problem is therefore not a ventilatory one. His target heart rate is = 151 bpm and he reaches 142 bpm (94% predicted). If the VO_2max is low and the patient reaches 80% of target heart rate, then the reason for a low VO_2max is a circulatory problem but we don't know if it is caused by

cardiovascular or pulmonary vascular disease. Arterial desaturation is more common in the latter and therefore this man has pulmonary vascular disease, probably as a result of pulmonary thromboembolic disease. Note that exercise desaturation also occurs in pulmonary diseases such as emphysema and fibrosing alveolitis.

101. B: Elevated CRP concentration

All the above are markers of active SLE disease except the raised c-reactive protein (CRP) concentration. The CRP is typically normal in active SLE. A raised CRP in a patient with SLE should raise the possibility of an associated infection. SLE as a disease is often controlled with variable doses of steroid, with or without other steroid-sparing/cytotoxic drugs such as azathioprine. This makes these patients prone to infection. Sometimes it is extremely difficult to differentiate between a flare-up of the disease or an infection.

102. C: There is a significant tendency for heavier ten-year-olds to have higher systolic blood pressures

The positive correlation indicates that there is a positive association between weight and systolic blood pressure (heavier people tend to have higher blood pressures). The P value shows that the association is significant (so C is correct). B may be correct but there is insufficient information given to conclude this. An interventional (rather than observational) study would be required to deduce whether A is correct. As the study is observational, a causal relationship cannot be inferred (D is incorrect). E is the least correct as the P value has been completely misinterpreted.

103. D: Loud, early pulmonary second sound

Pulmonary hypertension may result in right heart failure and an RV gallop but a gallop rhythm would occur earlier in left heart failure so D is a better answer. The increased pulmonary vascular resistance forces the pulmonary valve to shut early and loudly, later inducing pulmonary regurgitation as well.

A widely split second sound is a sign of systemic hypertension; fixed splitting and mid-systolic clicks are signs of atrial septal defect and mitral valve prolapse respectively. These are alternative causes of secondary pulmonary hypertension.

NB. the term 'primary pulmonary hypertension' is reserved for cases where no cause is identified.

104. B: Bioavailability following intravenous administration

Renal impairment can cause gastrointestinal oedema or uraemia, and both tend to impair drug absorption. Bioavailability after intravenous administration is always 100%. Drug distribution is altered by changes in fluid compartment volumes, and protein binding is altered due to hypoalbuminaemia. Hepatic metabolism and renal tubular secretion are both influenced by alterations in regional blood flow.

105. D: Intravenous amphotericin

The clinical findings suggest visceral leishmaniasis (kala-azar) caused by *Leishmania donovani*. The treatment of choice in the UK is amphotericin. (It was previously pentavalent antimony, or sodium stibogluconate.) Visceral leishmaniasis is currently a major problem in northern India and southern Sudan. HIV, disseminated TB and chronic malaria could all cause the same features, but massive splenomegaly is uncommon. Praziquantel is used for the treatment of helminth infections, such as schistosomiasis, in which massive splenomegaly is not seen.

106. C: Bullous pemphigoid

Bullous pemphigoid is a blistering disease of the elderly characterised by subepidermal blisters and positive immuno-fluorescence. It may be preceded by a history of pre-bullous itch and urticaria-like lesions. Pemphigoid gestationis (or herpes gestationis) is pemphigoid occurring in pregnancy; cicatricial pemphigoid presents with blisters and ulcers mainly affecting the mucosal membranes; dermatitis herpetiformis is a vesicular condition associated with gluten-sensitive enteropathy; pemphigus vulgaris demonstrates intra-epidermal, not subepidermal blisters.

107. D: Serum prolactin

The diagnosis not to miss is MEN type 1 (multiple endocrine neoplasia): remember the '3 P's' (pituitary, parathyroid, pancreas). Clues include the patient's young age (isolated primary hyperparathyroidism is much more common in postmenopausal women) and her family history. Her secondary amenorrhoea may be due to a prolactinoma.

108. E: Proliferative glomerulonephritis with 'full house' immunostaining

Haematuria, proteinuria and hypertension strongly suggest the elevated creatinine to be due to glomerulonephritis. The history, together with a positive ANA suggest a connective tissue disorder;

the normal CRP with elevated ESR makes lupus most likely. Renal biopsy appearances in lupus nephritis have been classified by WHO as follows:

Class 1 Normal
Class 2 Mesangial proliferative glomerulonephritis
Class 3 Focal and segmental proliferative glomerulonephritis
Class 4 Diffuse proliferative glomerulonephritis
Class 5 Membranous glomerulonephritis

The pathognomonic feature is deposition of all immunoglobulin classes (IgA, IgG and IgM) and complement (immunostaining most often performed for C1q) in the mesangium and glomerular capillary loops – 'full house' immunostaining. This immunostaining is an important feature, differentiatiating lupus nephritis from other causes of proliferative glomerulonephritis and subendothelial deposit formation. Mesangial IgA staining (in the absence of other immunoglobulins) is seen in IgA nephropathy. Necrotising glomerulonephritis with cellular crescent formation is most often seen in small vessel vasculitis. This is classically 'pauci-immune', i.e. there is no immunoglobulin or complement deposition. Proliferative glomerulonephritis with spikes on silver staining is diagnostic of membranous glomerulopathy.

109. C: Pyruvate kinase deficiency
Pyruvate kinase deficiency is an autosomal recessive disorder. It is caused by deficiency of the enzyme pyruvate kinase and thus failure to catalyse the conversion of phosphoenolpyruvate to pyruvate. This results in reduced adenosine triphosphate (ATP), the energy source of the red cell, and the red cells become rigid and are broken down. A large number of different defects of the gene encoding for pyruvate kinase have been described. Clinically, the level of anaemia varies between families. The patients have jaundice, gallstones and may have frontal bossing due to bone marrow hyperplasia. Splenectomy may alleviate the anaemia in some families. The blood film shows poikilocytosis and 'prickle' or 'sputnik' cells, particularly post-splenectomy

110. B: Detection of *C. difficile* toxin in the stool sample is diagnostic
C. difficile-associated colitis is primarily a nosocomial infection, reflecting the frequency of antibiotic use in hospitals as well as the widespread occurrence of the organism and its spores in the hospital environment. Antibiotic therapy disrupts the normal bacterial flora of the colon. Colonisation with *C. difficile* and release of toxins

cause mucosal inflammation. The organism itself is rarely invasive and colitis is mediated by toxins A and B, the latter being more potent. Although any antibiotic (with possible exceptions, such as streptomycin and vancomycin) may predispose to *C. difficile* infection, broad-spectrum antibiotics with activity against colonic bacteria, such as penicillins, cephalosporins and clindamycin, are common culprits, reflecting their widespread use.

Infection can range from asymptomatic carriage to fulminant colitis with perforation. Detection of *C. difficile* toxin is currently the most accurate test for the diagnosis of antibiotic-associated colitis. Anaerobic cultures to detect the organisms are expensive, take three to five days and detect non-toxicogenic strains, so are not specific for the diagnosis. Colonoscopy could reveal typical patchy, fibrinous, inflammatory exudates with pseudomembrane formation. However, rectal sparing occurs in up to one-third of cases. Rigid sigmoidoscopic examination of the rectum may therefore miss these lesions in a significant proportion of patients.

The first step in the management is to discontinue antibiotic therapy if possible. Specific therapy aimed at eradicating *C. difficile* is in those with severe or persistent symptoms. Metronidazole (oral or parenteral) and vancomycin (oral) are equally effective. Metronidazole is considered the drug of first choice because of concerns regarding the emergence of vancomycin resistant enterococci. Parenteral vancomycin is not significantly excreted into gut lumen, and so is not useful. Probiotics such as *Saccharomyces boulardii* and *Lactobacillus rhamnosus* GG have been used in refractory or recurrent infections.

111. E: A carotid Doppler should be performed
This quadrantanopia is not homonymous, so the lesion must lie anterior to the chiasm, i.e. in the retina or optic nerve. A branch retinal artery occlusion due to embolism is most likely.

112. B: Continuous history of adverse effects on society
Personality disorders consist of deeply ingrained maladaptive patterns of behaviour, present from adolescence and through adult life. As a consequence, either the patient or society is adversely affected. They should be distinguished from episodes of mental illness, which can present with abnormal behaviour, but which are confined to the episode of illness. Individuals with borderline personality disorders can experience pseudohallucinations. Individuals with antisocial personality disorders can be superficially charming, but have difficulty sustaining relationships and lack remorse.

113. E: Posterior inferior cerebellar artery

Ipsilateral Horner's syndrome and contralateral loss of pain and temperature sensation indicate damage in the dorsolateral region of the medulla – Wallenberg's syndrome. Lower vestibular nuclei are often involved, resulting in vertigo, vomiting and nystagmus; involvement of the inferior cerebellar peduncle will result in ipsilateral limb ataxia. This medullary syndrome is most often caused by occlusion of the posterior inferior cerebellar artery although, in some cases, an occlusion of the parent vertebral artery can be responsible.

114. D: Add a long-acting β$_2$-agonist

There is now very good evidence that the most appropriate step would be to add a long-acting β$_2$-agonist. The patient is currently on step 2 of the British Thoracic Society (BTS) asthma guidelines and moving to step 3 entails the addition of a long-acting β$_2$-agonist. Step 4 is now either high-dose inhaled steroids, oral theophylline, or an oral leukotriene receptor antagonist. Step 5 remains oral corticosteroids. Note that new BTS asthma guidelines were published February 2003.

115. D: Offer HIV testing

He is very likely to have multidrug resistant TB (resistance to at least rifampicin and isoniazid), now running at a high rate in eastern European prisons, particularly in parts of Russia. He should be started on a combination of at least five agents, three of which he has never had before, including one injectable agent. He should remain in isolation until he is shown (by sputum culture) to be non-infectious. Around 95% of rifampicin resistant strains can be detected by a single PCR, however there are multiple mutations involved in resistance to other agents. Isoniazid prophylaxis won't work if the organism is resistant. It is not clear what prophylaxis should be offered in these circumstances. HIV testing should now be offered to all UK TB patients.

116. A: Cardiac catheterisation

Cardiac catheterisation will reveal the culprit lesion and the available treatment options. Echocardiography will show any regional wall motion abnormality and the overall left ventricular function. Radionuclide perfusion imaging may also be required to clarify whether there is viable myocardium in apparent scar tissue to justify revascularising that region. The role of post-MI exercise testing is much diminished: it is still sometimes used in full-thickness

MI to detect ischaemic segments outside the infarct but its main role is in diagnosing stable angina and it has no logical role in acute coronary syndrome. Holter monitoring has no role in diagnosing ischaemia.

117. C: Keratoderma blennorrhagica

Reiter's syndrome is a reactive arthropathy typically seen in patients between 16 and 35. It may follow urethral tract infections or episodes of dysentery caused by *Salmonella*, *Shigella* or *Campylobacter* infection. There is a strong genetic association with HLA-B27. Conjunctivitis also commonly occurs. The skin manifestations include keratoderma blennorrhagica, circinate balanitis, oral aphthous ulceration and dystrophic nails.

118. A: Kimmelstiel-Wilson lesions

The history is typical of a patient with microvascular complications of diabetes mellitus, including diabetic nephropathy. The natural history of diabetic nephropathy is an initial 'silent phase' when the glomerular filtration rate is increased but there are no histopathological lesions, followed by development of microalbuminuria, frank proteinuria and, finally, impairment of excretory renal function. Once excretory renal function is abnormal, progression to end-stage renal failure is inevitable. At this stage, which is when many patients present, management focuses on slowing progression of the renal failure, which is achieved by control of hypertension, optimal glycaemic control, and treatment of hypercholesterolaemia. Hypertension should be treated with an angiotensin-converting enzyme inhibitor (ACEI) or an angiotensin-receptor antagonist if possible. If not tolerated, it is still essential to control blood pressure with whichever agents can be used. Hypercholesterolaemia should be treated with a statin as fibrates are associated with acclerated deterioration of renal function. Haematuria is frequently seen, and this may be a reason to proceed to renal biopsy in order to exclude other diagnoses.

119. C: Sick euthyroid syndrome

It is often better not to test thyroid function tests in acutely ill patients, unless possible hyper- or hypothyroidism is really considered to be contributing to their presentation. In the 'sick euthyroid syndrome', all parameters tend to 'droop' (TSH, FT4 and FT3). (There is debate about whether this condition should be treated: some authors advocate treatment, whilst others suggest that treatment does not improve the patient's prognosis, and may be harmful.) Remember that many of the symptoms of hyper- and hypothyroidism are non-specific, and may have other explanations (as in this case).

120. B: Urgent plasmapheresis

This patient has multiple myeloma, characterised by a neoplastic monoclonal proliferation of plasma cells in the bone marrow. Clinical features include bone pain and pathological fractures, anaemia, recurrent infections, abnormal bleeding tendency, renal failure and the hyperviscosity syndrome (characterised by central nervous system disturbance, visual disturbance and haemorrhages). This patient has typical features of hyperviscosity syndrome, both clinically and on laboratory indices. Treatment should therefore be urgent plasmapheresis. General resuscitative measures should also be introduced. Chemotherapy is required after the patient has been stabilised. It would be dangerous to transfuse this patient until the viscosity has been reduced.

121. E: Increased sodium absorption in the renal tubules

An elevated sinusoidal pressure is essential for the development of ascites, as fluid accumulation does not develop at a portal pressure gradient of less than 12 mmHg. However, ascites does not develop spontaneously in patients with portal vein thrombosis or non-cirrhotic causes of portal hypertension. Efflux of fluid from the sinusoidal space into the peritoneal cavity with increased production of hepatic lymph would be a self-limiting process once the intravascular space becomes depleted. However, formation of ascites is a continuous process, with constant replenishment of intravascular volume. Sodium and water retention is critical in the pathogenesis of ascites in the presence of portal hypertension. Sodium handling is abnormal in patients with cirrhosis, even in the pre-ascitic stage.

Aldosterone plays a major role, since it increases sodium retention in the distal tubules. Even in the presence of normal aldosterone levels renal sensitivity to aldosterone may be enhanced in cirrhosis. The underlying cause of activation of sodium-retaining pathways is still disputed.

A unifying hypothesis, known as the 'vasodilatation hypothesis' was put forward to explain the known observations with regard to the development of salt-retaining states. According to this, systemic vasodilatation present in cirrhosis leads to a decrease in 'effective' blood volume and to activation of the renin-angiotensin-aldosterone system and the sympathetic nervous system, which leads to sodium and water retention.

122. D: Prosopagnosia

Prosopagnosia is associated with damage to the fusiform gyrus (occipitotemporal cortex). Dyspraxias and body image disorders are associated with parietal lobe dysfunction. These include autotopagnosia – the inability to recognise parts of the body, as well as anosognosia – a lack of awareness of disease. Right–left disorientation can occur in dominant parietal lobe problems.

123. A: Increase the inspired oxygen

The most important thing to do in these circumstances is to increase the PaO_2 – otherwise he will die from hypoxaemia. Although increasing the FiO_2 may result in worsening hypercapnia, one cannot leave this man with such a low oxygen level. Should the $PaCO_2$ increase, then it is appropriate to use non-invasive ventilation, if available. BiPAP would be better than CPAP in patients with COPD as the expiratory pressure may be set at a lower level than the inspiratory pressure, thus enabling the patient to exhale more easily. If the expiratory pressure is too high, then COPD patients find it difficult to breathe out against the machine and this can result in worsening gas trapping with hyperinflation. If non-invasive ventilation (NIV) is not available, then the intravenous stimulant doxapram may be of short-term use. Intubation could also be used as the patient has a reversible cause for his acute deterioration but NIV, if available, is preferable.

124. C: Guillain-Barré syndrome

Back pain is a common early feature of Guillain-Barré syndrome, and may lead to misdiagnosis. Guillain-Barré syndrome is an acute demyelinating polyneuropathy characterised by progressive weakness (often ascending), areflexia and characteristic findings on nerve conduction studies/EMG. In about one-third of patients the disorder is preceded by an infection.

125. C: Plain X-ray of the skull

Paget's disease of bone is a focal disorder of bone remodelling characterised by an increase in the number and size of osteoclasts in affected skeletal sites while the rest of the skeleton is spared.

Diagnosis of Paget's disease may be suspected based on the symptoms, but radiographs are the most specific diagnostic test. The lesions are clearly demarcated and confined to individual bones.

Radiographs include both lytic (early) and sclerotic (late) findings. Patchy areas of increased radiolucency are characteristic of the osteolytic stage. Classically, the osteolytic patches are circumscribed (osteoporosis circumscripta). The sclerotic phase is characterised by increased bone density. The bones are enlarged and irregular with coarse trabeculation. New bone may impinge on the medulla from the cortex (cotton wool appearance).

Many patients are diagnosed incidentally in the asymptomatic phase by plain radiographs that show localised enlargement of bone. These radiographs often have a high specificity because of their classic nature, but a low sensitivity. Isotope bone scans can be used to increase the sensitivity in patients suspected of having Paget's disease; however, the bone scan is less specific and should be interpreted cautiously. Isotope bone scans are useful in assessing disease activity and monitoring response to treatment. Once a diagnosis of Paget's disease is confirmed, repeat radiographs are required only to monitoring degeneration around weight-bearing joints. Computed tomography and magnetic resonance imaging have little place in the evaluation of Paget's disease.

126. B: Capture and fusion beats

Capture beats (a normal complex captured in a string of abnormal complexes) and fusion beats (a complex beginning with tachycardic morphology but finishing with normal morphology) are diagnostic of ventricular tachycardia (VT). VT may be of left bundle branch block or right bundle branch block morphology but there is often concordance across the chest leads, and a broader QRS complex favours VT over aberrant conduction.

127. E: Hydrocortisone

An old 'endocrine chestnut': the hydrocortisone should be started first. If thyroxine is started first (which can happen inadvertently if the diagnosis of hypocortisolism is not suspected) you may precipitate an addisonian crisis. Also remember that fludrocortisone is not needed if the problem is in the pituitary (lack of ACTH) rather than in the adrenal (e.g. autoimmune Addison's disease). Mineralocorticoid activity is regulated by the renin-angiotensin-aldosterone system.

128. B: Immune reconstitution illness

As a patient's immune system starts to improve on antiretroviral therapy (partly manifested by a rise in CD4 count), previously ignored immune targets are recognised. It is not uncommon for the site of mycobacterial infection to develop an inflammatory reaction. Previously unrecognised mycobacterial nodes may enlarge and ulcerate if situated subcutaneously, even though the mycobacteria may have been killed by appropriate therapy. The clinical findings are also compatible with lymphoma, but the timing is typical of an immune reconstitution syndrome. Extrapulmonary *Pneumocystis* is rare and usually affects the liver and spleen. *Cryptococcus* can cause a pneumonia and infiltrate the liver and spleen. Cytomegalovirus problems occur through reactivation and are not associated with lymphadenopathy.

129. E: Infusion of factor IX concentrate

Haemophilia B or Christmas disease is an X-linked disorder characterised by deficiency of factor IX. The clinical features are similar to haemophilia A, with joint bleeding and prolonged bleeding after trauma or surgery. It is five times less common than haemophilia A. Laboratory tests show a prolonged APTT and decreased factor IX level with factor IX clotting assays. Bleeding episodes are treated with factor IX concentrates. Recombinant factor IX is now available. Treatment is usually only required once a day as factor IX concentrates have a longer half-life than factor VIII concentrates.

130. B: Interstitial nephritis

Non-steroidal anti-inflammatory drugs (NSAIDs) may cause renal 'disease' in three ways:

- They reduce glomerular filtration pressure and therefore the glomerular filtration rate by preventing prostaglandin-mediated dilatation of the glomerular afferent arteriole. This is part of the normal autoregulatory function of the glomerulus. In normal individuals this physiological effect will not cause significant impairment of excretory renal function. However, in a patient whose renal function is compromised, this effect may be significant. It is particularly important if ACEI or angiotensin-receptor antagonists are co-administered as these agents prevent the second autoregulatory mechanism (efferent arteriolar vasoconstriction).
- Indometacin is rarely associated with minimal change nephropathy.
- NSAIDs are a common cause of interstitial nephritis.

There is nothing in the history to suggest lupus nephritis. Although membranous nephropathy would typically present with heavy proteinuria and renal function is often normal at presentation, it cannot be explained by the previous orthopaedic procedure and alternative explanations are therefore preferred. Acute tubular necrosis can occur after any operation if prolonged hypotension is seen. It is more likely if nephrotoxic drugs, such as aminoglycosides, are co-administered. This is unlikely after a routine orthopaedic procedure and would present immediately postop. As above, indometacin-induced minimal change nephropathy is possible. However, by far the most likely diagnosis is indometacin-induced interstitial nephritis. The diagnosis would be confirmed by renal biopsy. With withdrawal of the indometacin, recovery of normal renal function and resolution of proteinuria would be expected. Steroids may speed recovery and may be of use in patients with very heavy proteinuria. They do not affect the prognosis.

131. B: Langerhans cell histiocytosis

There are not many causes of flitting multifocal consolidation but you should remember the following five causes: commonly, cryptogenic organising pneumonia, allergic bronchopulmonary aspergillosis, eosinophilic pneumonia; less commonly, sarcoidosis, acute extrinsic allergic alveolitis. Langerhans cell histiocytosis, a disease of cigarette smokers, is characterised by pulmonary nodules that cavitate, giving rise to cystic changes.

132. C: Small bowel contrast studies should be performed to look for ileal Crohn's disease

This clinical presentation, with diarrhoea, abdominal pain with signs and investigations suggestive of an inflammatory process is highly suggestive of Crohn's disease. Oral aphthoid ulcers are recognised features of Crohn's disease and the ileocaecal region is commonest site involved. The long duration of the symptoms and the history of persistent diarrhoea make appendicitis an unlikely diagnosis. *Yersinia* enterocolitis can mimic Crohn's disease and must be excluded using paired serology. Behçet's disease is characterised by recurrent orogenital ulcerations, uveitis, synovitis, occlusive venulitis, and meningoencephalitis. The right colon is the commonest gastrointestinal site to be involved in ulceration in Behçet's disease and perforation is one of the causes of mortality in this group of patients. Ulcerative colitis involves the large bowel (although backwash ileitis is recognised) and so presents with bloody diarrhoea. Abdominal pain is a less common feature of ulcerative colitis and occurs in patients with acute severe colitis.

133. D: Marginal erosions

Radiographs can provide objective evidence of the disease. Findings consistent with osteoarthritis include the presence of joint-space narrowing, osteophyte formation, pseudocysts in subchondral bone, and increased density of subchondral bone.

In general, radiographic evidence of bone erosions and juxta-articular osteoporosis are consistent with inflammatory arthropathy rather than osteoarthritis.

134. A: Anterior spinal artery occlusion

The anterior spinal artery and its branches supply the anterior two-thirds of the spinal cord, with the posterior spinal artery supplying the posterior third. Vascular thrombosis is uncommon and compression (e.g. tumours or acute disc prolapse) or occlusion (e.g. dissecting aneurysm) are more common causes of infarction. Sudden pain in the back in the distribution of the affected segment is associated with bilateral flaccid weakness. The sensory loss is dissociated, with impaired pinprick and temperature sensation below the level of the infarct, while touch, proprioception and vibration sense are typically spared because they are conducted in the posterior columns.

135. D: He should inform the DVLA and may resume driving a private vehicle after one month if passed fit but will be required to complete three stages of the Bruce protocol off anti-anginals and without evidence of ischaemia to regain LGV entitlement

Following myocardial infarction, a patient should refrain from driving for one month and it is good practice for them to be seen in Outpatients or by the GP to pass them fit to drive a private vehicle. LGV and PCV rules are much stricter: patients must complete three stages of the Bruce protocol without ischaemic changes, having been off anti-anginals for 48 hours. They may then be issued with a short-term (three-year) licence. Information on licensing in medical conditions is available on the DVLA website (www.dvla.gov.uk/at_a_glance/content.htm).

136. E: BMI may be a confounder – it should be corrected for in the analysis

E is the correct answer. D is the next nearest correct, but the data does not need to be dichotomised into low and high BMI in order to investigate whether BMI is a confounder. Dichotomising will lose information and it is preferable to leave as a continuum. Similarly, A may help in the interpretation but we do not know how many are affected and whether this action will remove the problem. If we were sure that BMI was not associated with blood pressure, then B would be correct. C is incorrect because differences in the BMI distribution are known to have occurred by chance, despite randomisation.

137. E: Stevens-Johnson syndrome
Erythromycin enhances the concentrations of the polypeptide motilin, which increases gastric emptying and small bowel propulsion (due to hepatic enzyme inhibition). Although erythromycin can increase the corrected QT interval (QTc), this is not usually of clinical significance. Stevens-Johnson syndrome has been reported with sulphonamide use, including co-trimoxazole.

138. B: Atenolol
There are a number of drugs which can exacerbate psoriasis, including β-blockers, lithium carbonate and antimalarials. The withdrawal of oral steroids can also cause this.

139. A: Start treatment with meropenem and gentamicin prior to identification of the organism
Standard 'blind' therapy for endocarditis is with benzylpenicillin and gentamicin unless the patient is penicillin-allergic, when vancomycin and gentamicin are recommended. *Streptococcus bovis* endocarditis is associated with carcinoma of the colon. Two weeks' treatment is recommended for uncomplicated, fully sensitive *S. viridans* or *S. bovis* infections. Recurrent embolic phenomena are an indication for urgent surgical intervention.

140. A: Renal vein thrombosis
Patients with heavy proteinuria are at increased risk of venous thrombosis, with renal vein thrombosis being seen in such patients. This presents with loin pain, haematuria and increase in the protein leak, and deterioration of excretory renal function. Diagnosis can be made by Doppler ultrasound. The usual precipitant to sloughing of the renal papillae is hypotension. Conditions predisposing to this include diabetic nephropathy, analgesic nephropathy and sickle cell anaemia. It usually occurs unilaterally and only causes deterioration in excretory renal function if there is already significant impairment. Although any drug could potentially cause interstitial nephritis, it is not common with statins. Approximately 5% of renal biopsies are complicated by perinephric or intrarenal haemorrhage. Perinephric haemorrhage may cause pain but would present within 48 hours. It is very unlikely to cause deterioration of excretory renal function. Life-threatening haemorrahage is a recognized complication, death due

to renal biopsy occurring in approximately 0.1% of biopsies. Dipstick haematuria is frequently seen post-biopsy. Heavy bleeding may be associated with frank haematuria and if clot retention results, excretory renal function may deteriorate. Again, this would present soon after biopsy. Any type of glomerulonephritis can undergo acute crescentic change, which is diagnosed by cellular crescent formation on renal biopsy. This is associated with dipstick haematuria and proteinuria, and deterioration of excretory renal function. It is uncommon and would not classically be associated with loin pain.

141. C: She should be converted from tablets to insulin therapy
All of the advice is sound, but you should prioritise conversion of all pregnant patients with type 2 diabetes from oral hypoglycaemic agents to insulin therapy. Although some recent studies suggest oral hypoglycaemic agents may be used in pregnancy, there is still general concern about their safety, and most patients are treated with insulin (often as a qds 'basal bolus' regimen). Extremely tight glycaemic control improves the outcome of diabetic pregnancies, but does increase the risk of hypoglycaemia, and this should be discussed with patients and their partners. Retinopathy may worsen in pregnancy, so retinal screening is imperative, with referral to an ophthalmologist if indicated.

142. C: Patient's age is a factor predicting a poor prognosis without liver transplantation
Aetiology is the most important variable predicting survival in acute hepatic failure.

The most common cause of acute liver failure in the UK is paracetamol toxicity, followed by seronegative hepatitis (non-A to non-E hepatitis), hepatitis B, idiosyncratic drug reactions, and hepatitis A. The selection of patients for transplantation in acute liver failure is based on predictive models. Those fulfilling the King's College Hospital criteria have less than a 10% chance of survival without liver transplantation. For paracetamol-related acute hepatic failure, a blood pH <7.30 despite adequate fluid resuscitation, or the combination of prothrombin time (PT) >100 s and creatinine >300 μmol/l with grade 3 or 4 encephalopathy, are indications for transplantation. Indications for liver transplantation in non-paracetamol-related cases, are a PT >100 s, regardless of degree of encephalopathy, or any three of the following:

1. Aetiology: non-A non-B hepatitis or idiosyncratic drug reactions
2. Age <10 or >40 years

3. Jaundice to encephalopathy interval of more than seven days
4. Prothrombin time >50 s
5. Serum bilirubin >300 μmol/l

143. B: Ham's test

Paroxysmal nocturnal haemoglobinuria (PNH) is a rare acquired clonal disorder of stem cells where there is deficient production of the glycosyl-phosphatidylinositol (GPI) anchor which attaches proteins to the cell surface. Patients have acquired mutations of the phosphatidylinositol glycan protein (PIG-A) gene on the X chromosome. Patients present with anaemia and thrombocytopenia, and intravascular haemolysis which causes haemoglobinuria and haemosiderinuria. Thrombosis is another prominent feature. The diagnosis is made using Ham's test where red cell lysis is demonstrated at low pH. Flow cytometry will demonstrate the loss of expression of GPI-linked proteins such as CD55 and CD59. The bone marrow is usually hypoplastic and the PNH clone may expand as a result of a selective pressure, i.e. it may occur as a result of an episode of aplasia.

144. C: Diazepam

Multiple sclerosis is associated with a high risk of developing clinical depression. Unfortunately, several of the treatments used in multiple sclerosis can increase the risk of developing depression. Diazepam can be used to treat muscle spasms. It has an effect on mood symptoms, in particular anxiety. Diazepam is unlikely to produce depression.

145. C: Ulnar nerve

Sensory supply to the little finger is from the dorsal cutaneous branch of the ulnar nerve. The C8–T1 components of the ulnar nerve are motor to the dorsal interossei, which abduct the fingers (palmar interossei adduct – 'pad and dab' are the mnemonics to remember). The most likely site for ulnar nerve damage is at the elbow.

146. B: Rifampicin and isoniazid

MDRTB is defined as resistance to rifampicin and isoniazid, with/without resistance to other drugs. It can be primary (contact with an MDRTB patient) or secondary (initially drug-susceptible TB that becomes MDRTB through either non-compliance or inadequate treatment regimen). One should treat MDRTB by starting at least five drugs to which the mycobacteria are likely to be sensitive and modify according to sensitivities. Expert advice is always required and **never add a single drug to a failing regimen** as this favours the development of resistance to that drug. Therefore, always add combinations of two to three drugs at a time. Treatment is usually required for long periods of time, i.e. 18–24 months. Notification to the Public Health Laboratory is mandatory.

147. D: Tophus of the ear

Treatment of gout depends on its stage of progression. In patients with asymptomatic hyperuricaemia and acute intermittent gout (occurring fewer than three times per year), long-term management consists of modification of risk factors (i.e. avoidance of diuretics and alcohol, weight loss, and avoidance of dehydration). These measures may all reduce gout attacks by lowering uric acid levels. Indications for uric acid-lowering therapy include tophaceous gout, frequent attacks (three or more per year) and urate nephropathy. Non-steroidal anti-inflammatory drugs (NSAIDs) work well in cases of acute gout, but they should not be used in clinical settings in which a patient is at high risk for NSAID complications. In such a patient, intra-articular injection is the safest treatment and has the added benefit of a rapid decrease in pain. Aspiration alone is helpful because removal of crystal-laden fluid can down-regulate the inflammatory process. Although joints previously involved in gout attacks have a higher likelihood of becoming affected, the presence of more than one affected joint makes this possibility very unlikely. More recently, selective cyclo-oxygenase-2 inhibitors such as etoricoxib have been used as alternative treatment to traditional NSAIDs for acute gout.

148. B: Parvovirus B19

The rash and arthritis of parvovirus B19 infection are immunologically mediated and occur a few days after the viraemia and fever. Fever is usually present in rubella and rheumatic fever at this stage. HHV-6 is acquired by > 90% of the population by the age of three years, so adult acute HHV-6 infection is extremely rare. The gonococcus does not produce a reticular rash.

149. C: Male sex, hypertension and renal impairment at presentation are poor prognostic indicators

The history is of a young adult man presenting with nephrotic syndrome. He has no pre-existing illness and there has been no drug exposure and no intercurrent illness. Glomerulonephritis (GN) is therefore the likely cause. Statistically, the four most likely histological diagnoses are: minimal change nephropathy (83% of children and 28% of adults), membranous glomerulonephropathy (1% of children and 25% of adults), focal segmental glomerulosclerosis (8% of children and 15% of adults) and mesangiocapillary glomerulonephritis (5% of children and 12% of adults). For all of these, prognosis is affected adversely by male sex, hypertension and renal impairment at presentation. An underlying malignancy is found in 4–11% of patients with membranous glomerulonephritis, almost all such patients being over the age of 50. In most (70–75%), the malignancy is evident at the time of diagnosis. The renal biopsy in membranous GN demonstrates sub-epithelial deposits and the association is with hepatitis B, not hepatitis C.

150. D: Peripheral neuropathy
Amiodarone has widespread toxicity. Hyperthyroid reactions require the stopping of the drug but hypothyroid reactions can be managed with thyroxine replacement. Patients on amiodarone should have regular assessments of liver and thyroid biochemistry. Of the above listed effects, corneal deposits are reversible on stopping the drug, peripheral neuropathy may reverse, but lung and liver damage often have an irreversible element. The slate-grey pigmentation is also persistent.

151. E: Sodium valproate
Aspirin confers a risk of Reye's syndrome. Carbimazole is capable of causing neonatal goitre and/or hypothyroidism. The newborn has increased sensitivity to benzodiazepines, which can result in lethargy and respiratory depression. Tetracyclines are taken up into developing bones and teeth, and can cause dental discoloration. Other drugs that should be avoided include barbiturates (drowsiness) and amiodarone (neonatal hypothyroidism). Other drugs that are generally regarded as safe include penicillins, theophylline, sodium valproate, carbamazepine, phenytoin, β-blockers, warfarin and heparin.

152. C: Barium enema would be useful to look for megacolon
Streaky rectal bleeding with painful defaecation suggests acute anal fissure associated with severe constipation. Barium enema showing a narrowed segment in the recto-sigmoid area with massive dilatation above is typical of Hirschsprung's disease. Chronic idiopathic megacolon is characterised by: onset in late childhood; severe chronic constipation; faecal loading palpable on digital examination

of the rectum; and barium enema studies showing the entire colon distended with stools. Using physiological studies, patients with severe idiopathic constipation may be categorised into three subgroups, including 1) slow-transit constipation, 2) pelvic floor dysfunction and 3) undefined. Colonic transit studies using radio-opaque markers provide useful information, identifying those with slow transit. Pelvic floor dyssynergia is associated with failure of the puborectalis and external anal sphincter muscles to relax during attempted defaecation. Pelvic floor dyssynergia is suggested by symptoms of straining at defaecation or a feeling of incomplete evacuation. Colonic transit may show recto-sigmoid delay. Anorectal manometry with an anal sphincter electromyogram (EMG) would be able to demonstrate the pathophysiological changes. In addition, the presence of internal anal sphincter relaxation in response to rectal distension excludes the diagnosis of Hirschsprung's disease in children and adults with lifelong constipation, especially in the presence of megarectum. Defaecography has a number of limitations and abnormalities such as rectocele are common in the population, being of uncertain significance. Constipation of undefined aetiology occurs in a heterogeneous group of patients, although there is no evidence to support the view that most of these patients have irritable bowel syndrome.

153. E: Lichen planus

The Koebner phenomenon describes the induction of skin lesions by, and at the site of, trauma such as scratch marks or operative incisions. Causes of the Koebner phenomenon are psoriasis, lichen planus, vitiligo, viral warts, molluscum contagiosum and bullous pemphigoid.

154. D: 24-hour urine collection for catecholamines

The patient may have a phaeochromocytoma. The urinary free catecholamines assay has superceded the urinary VMA assay, as it is less influenced by components of the patient's diet. Urinary 5-HIAA is increased in carcinoid syndrome. Again, remember to make the biochemical diagnosis before scanning the patient. Once the diagnosis has been made, the phaeochromocytoma can be localised using a CT scan of the abdomen and an MIBG radioisotope scan.

155. D: Anti-centromere antibodies are diagnostic for CREST syndrome

There are two main types of scleroderma:

- One type is localised scleroderma, which affects mainly the skin, for example 'morphea'.

- The other type is systemic sclerosis (SSc), affecting the skin as well as the internal organs, such as the heart, lungs and kidneys.

The systemic form is subdivided into limited cutaneous systemic sclerosis (CREST) and diffuse cutaneous SSc. Scleroderma literally means 'hard skin'. However, there is a third type of SSc that presents no skin involvement and only involves the internal organs, such as the heart, lungs and kidneys. This is called 'scleroderma sine scleroderma'. This means, literally, 'scleroderma without scleroderma', which refers to scleroderma without the skin involvement. Subcutaneous calcification (calcinosis) is not unique for the limited type and is also common in the diffuse form of SSc.

There is no known cure for scleroderma. The five-year survival rate is 80–85%. No treatment has been scientifically proved to alter the overall course of the disease. Anti-centromere (kinetochore) antibodies are directed against components of the mitotic spindle apparatus. They are specific for limited systemic sclerosis (CREST syndrome) which comprise the following features: Raynaud's phenomenon, oesophageal dysmotility, sclerodactyly, telangiectasias and limited cutaneous involvement. Anti-topoisomerase-I (Scl-70) antibodies are associated with generalised skin involvement in patients with diffuse SSc, where there is higher incidence of pulmonary fibrosis, cardiac involvement and digital pitting scars. They are regarded as diagnostic for diffuse systemic sclerosis but can only be identified in 30% of cases.

156. B: Warfarin

This patient has atrial fibrillation (AF) in association with transient ischaemic attacks (TIAs). The priority is anticoagulation to prevent further cerebrovascular events. Aspirin is less appropriate given the recurrent events and the presence of atrial fibrillation. Digoxin controls the rate of AF but will not restore the heart to sinus rhythm; in this case the rate is already acceptably controlled. As he is haemodynamically stable, DC cardioversion would only be appropriate if the AF was of recent onset, which is unlikely in view of the previous TIAs. Note that elective cardioversion would require prior anticoagulation in any case.

157. E: Haemoglobin H disease

Haemoglobin H disease is due to the deletion of three out of the four α-chain globin genes. Clinical features are variable but patients have moderate anaemia and jaundice due to the haemolysis. Most patients have hepatosplenomegaly and, frequently, chronic leg ulceration. The patients have a microcytic anaemia, polychromasia, target cells and NRBC on the blood film. Brilliant cresyl-blue staining shows 'golf ball' inclusions or Hb H inclusions, which are tetramers of β-chains which have polymerised due to lack of α-chain globin genes. Haemoglobin electrophoresis detects the HbH. Haemoglobin H disease is a form of thalassaemia intermedia. Treatment is not usually required.

158. A: High-dose systemic steroids
The emergency treatment of sight-threatening dysthyroid eye disease is initially with high-dose systemic steroids. Only if this fails should surgical decompression be contemplated. Radiotherapy takes several weeks to be effective.

159. A: Rectal biopsy
He has acute Katayama fever due to schistosomiasis acquired a few weeks previously. Diagnosis can usually be made by looking for eggs in a rectal biopsy. Stool examination is less sensitive. A slit skin smear is used to diagnose multibacillary leprosy and cutaneous leishmaniasis. Strongyloidiasis can cause a marked eosinophilia with rapidly migratory small patches of urticaria.

160. B: Agranulocytosis
Clozapine is the only antipsychotic that has been demonstrated to have superior efficacy in treatment-resistant schizophrenia. It has a lesser effect on dopamine receptors than typical antipsychotics. It is therefore less likely to produce extrapyramidal side effects such as dystonic reactions, or elevated prolactin levels and resultant galactorrhoea, amenorrhoea or impotence. The 1% risk of agranulocytosis requires regular blood monitoring and limits a more widespread use of the medication.

161. C: CD4 count of 350 cells/μl is a contraindication to curative resection
Observational studies have revealed that lung cancer is increased 3–4 times in the HIV-positive population. Adenocarcinoma is the commonest type and accounts for 45–50% cases. TNM status is independent of the CD4 count and therefore the CD4 count is not used to exclude surgery. Compared to non-HIV patients, HIV-positive patients have usually smoked more cigarettes (40/day vs. 20/day), present younger (38 vs. 53 years), and have a worse median survival (5 vs. 10 months).

162. A: It is probably due to vasculitis if there is circulating anti-neutrophil cytoplasmic antibody (ANCA) present

The history of renal impairment, hypertension, haematuria and proteinuria is strongly suggestive of glomerulonephritis. As is often the case at presentation, no definitive information is given to decide if this is acute, acute on chronic, or chronic renal failure. However, the history and purpuric rash are strongly suggestive of small vessel vasculitis causing rapidly progressive glomerulonephritis (RPGN). An ultrasound scan should be performed urgently to exclude obstruction due to malignancy and determine renal size and echogenicity. If the renal size is normal the diagnosis of acute renal failure secondary to rapidly progressive glomerulonephritis is supported and a renal biopsy should be performed. The presence of high titres of anti-PR3 or anti-MPO antibodies (ANCA) would strongly support the diagnosis of RPGN secondary to small vessel vasculitis. If this diagnosis is confirmed, treatment should be with oral cyclophosphamide and corticosteroids. Plasma exchange is indicated in patients who are dialysis-dependent or who have a plasma creatinine > 500 μmol/l. Haemoptysis is not confined to antiglomerular basement membrane (anti-GMB) disease, being common in both Wegener's granulomatosis and microscopic polyarteritis. Anti-GBM disease is a rare diagnosis, Wegener's granulomatosis or microscopic polyarteritis being much more likely. For patients who are not dialysis-dependent at presentation, significant recovery of renal function would be expected. Mesangiocapillary glomerulonephritis may occur as a paraneoplastic lesion and would present in a similar manner with echogenic, small kidneys on ultrasound. Type 2 mesangiocapillary GN is associated with circulating nephritic factor.

163. A: Change in bowel habit

The best guide to digoxin toxicity is symptoms, which are often vague but gastrointestinal complaints are common. Persistent atrial fibrillation is common in PAF treated with digoxin because it is not effective at maintaining sinus rhythm. The 'reverse tick' effect is a result of digoxin therapy but does not indicate toxicity. Right axis deviation is not a sign of digoxin toxicity. Ventricular ectopics are normal although they increase in digoxin toxicity.

164. C: Family history of adult polycystic kidney disease

Both subarachnoid haemorrhage and bacterial meningitis are neurological emergencies, and both computed tomography and lumbar puncture are required (with intravenous antibiotic cover until meningitis is excluded). Diabetes, opiate misuse and migraine are not ordinarily risk factors for either condition. Adult polycystic kidney disease has autosomal dominant inheritance and 25% will have berry aneurysms, with about half of those succumbing to subarachnoid haemorrhage at some point.

165. **C: Inhibition of thromboxane A$_2$ synthesis by platelets**
Aspirin irreversibly inhibits cyclo-oxygenase. In platelets, this prevents generation of the pro-aggregatory prostaglandin TXA$_2$. Platelets are anucleate and, therefore, recovery of function depends on synthesis of new platelets and takes around 10–12 days. Low dosages of aspirin used for thromboprophylaxis (75–150 mg) do not have analgesic effects, which require significantly higher doses (1–4 g/day). Low doses can inhibit active tubular secretion, thereby reducing urate clearance and promoting the risk of acute gout. Aspirin does not alter coagulation.

166. **C: Multiple staphylococcal abscesses**
The history is most compatible with an acute bacteraemic or septicaemic illness, making bacterial brain abscesses the most likely. (Other common bacterial causes are *Streptococcus milleri*-group organisms, anaerobes and mixed infections.) Toxoplasmosis, tuberculomas and cysticercosis (*Taenia saginata*, pork tapeworm) do not present as very acute febrile illnesses. HSV encephalitis does not lead to abscess formation, but causes MMR changes in the temporal and frontal lobes.

167. **C: Oesophageal carcinoma**
Tylosis (palmar/plantar keratoderma) is associated with oesophageal carcinoma. Acute myeloid leukaemia is associated with Sweet's syndrome (acute febrile neutrophilic dermatosis); bronchial carcinoma is associated with erythema gyratum repens and dermatomyositis; lymphoma is associated with acquired ichthyosis; glucagonoma is associated with necrolytic migratory erythema.

168. **B: Mesangial IgA disease**
In a fit young patient, microscopic haematuria together with macroscopic haematuria during times of intercurrent illness is strongly suggestive of mesangial IgA disease (IgA nephropathy). Infection, calculi and tumours should be excluded. Henoch-Schönlein syndrome refers specifically to haematuria occurring in the context of a purpuric rash, usually preceded by abdominal pain. Renal biopsy demonstrates pathology indistinguishable from that

seen in IgA disease. The history is not that of Henoch-Schönlein syndrome. There is no history to explain the development of either acute tubular necrosis or rhabdomyolysis, neither of which would cause haematuria. Rhabdomyolysis will cause dark urine due to myoglobinuria. Membranous nephropathy classically presents with proteinuria and almost never causes haematuria.

169. A: Give 0.5 mg vitamin K intravenously

The management of warfarin overdosage as advised by the British Society for Haematology and quoted in the *British National Formulary* is follows:

- Major bleeding: stop warfarin; give 5 mg of vitamin K intravenously; give prothrombin complex concentrate 50 units/kg or, if not available, fresh frozen plasma 15 ml/kg.
- INR > 8.0, no bleeding or minor bleeding: stop warfarin and restart when INR < 5.0; if there are other risk factors for bleeding give 0.5 mg vitamin K intravenously or 5 mg orally.
- INR 6.0–8.0, no bleeding or minor bleeding: stop warfarin and restart when INR < 5.0.
- INR < 6.0 but more than 0.5 units above the target value: reduce or stop warfarin; restart when INR < 5.0.
- Unexpected bleeding at therapeutic levels: always investigate the possibility of an underlying cause, e.g. unsuspected renal or gastrointestinal pathology.

170. A: Estimation of hepatic copper concentration is the definitive test to establish the diagnosis of Wilson's disease

Wilson's disease is inherited as an autosomal recessive or co-dominant disease. The abnormal gene is on chromosome 13 at the *ATP7B* site. The gene product is a copper-translocating P-type ATPase. The defective liver-specific transporter is unable to transport copper into bile adequately, leading to accumulation of copper in liver and other tissues. Heterozygotes with a single mutation do not develop any manifestations of the disease, although there may be minimal abnormalities in copper parameters, suggesting the pattern of inheritance as co-dominant, with one normal allele sufficient to prevent the development of the disease. Several polymorphisms in the *ATP7B* gene have been described. All-inclusive genotyping is not available and if a specific mutation is identified in the patient, this could be used in screening the siblings.

Kayser-Fleischer rings are invariably present in patients who have neurological manifestations, but may be absent in those with hepatic manifestations only. About 5% of homozygotes have a normal caeruloplasmin level. Patients with acute liver failure due to Wilson's disease present with a normal caeruloplasmin level, consistent with the acute phase reactant nature of the protein. Urinary copper excretion is elevated in patients as a result of increased renal clearance of circulating free copper. This is not widely used as a clinical test, but may be useful in identifying those who are non-compliant with penicillamine treatment. The liver copper concentration is the definitive test to establish the diagnosis of Wilson's disease. Care must be taken to obtain and store the liver sample in copper-free containers. A liver copper level above 250 μg/g dry weight is diagnostic.

171. B: Body image distortion

Key features of bulimia nervosa include a constant preoccupation with food, accompanied by episodes of overeating (bingeing). Patients attempt to counteract the fattening effect of food, for example with periods of starvation or vomiting. Patients have a fear of fatness. Body image distortion is present in anorexia nervosa and involves a patient believing they are fat when they are very underweight.

172. C: Transdiaphragmatic pressure measurement

The history described is classic of someone with bilateral diaphragm weakness. The reason for being worse when standing vertically in water is that there is a greater column of water exerting pressure on the abdominal contents, which are displaced superiorly. When the patient starts swimming he changes position to horizontal and therefore the column of water exerting pressure on the abdomen is decreased. Respiratory muscle strength may be assessed with mouth pressures: maximum inspiratory pressure (**MIP**) is taken from residual volume and should normally be at least -80 **cmH$_2$O**; maximum expiratory pressure (**MEP**) is taken from total lung capacity and should normally be at least $+80$ **cmH$_2$O**. Diaphragmatic strength can be measured by using pressure balloons, one in the oesophagus and one in the stomach. Sniff $P_{di} = P_{gas} - P_{oes}$, which should normally be > 100 cmH$_2$O in men and > 80 cmH$_2$O in women. A decreased P_{di} implies diaphragm weakness/paralysis.

173. C: Ferritin level

In patients with osteoarthritis laboratory tests are generally normal, including the ESR. The indications for laboratory tests in osteoarthritis are to exclude secondary causes of osteoarthritis, including metabolic diseases and the endocrinopathies. In this case, the factors that suggest a possible secondary cause of osteoarthritis are the relatively young age of the patient, who does not have an occupational risk for premature osteoarthritis, and the unusual distribution involving the metacarpals. Abnormalities of the second and third metacarpal joints are a classic sign of haemochromatosis. The mechanism of damage in haemochromatosis is believed to be direct damage to chondrocytes by iron ions.

174. C: Propranolol

This woman has essential tremor. This is a 6–8 Hz tremor, typically of the hands but also affecting other body parts (in particular the head, legs, trunk and voice). It is the most common adult neurological disorder, with a prevalence twenty times that of Parkinson's disease. Genetic factors play a major role, with 60–80% patients reporting a family history; the gene is unknown, but inheritance is autosomal dominant. Worsened by posture and stress, the tremor is improved by rest, alcohol and β-blockers. Propranolol is therefore the most appropriate initial treatment for her condition. Primidone is also effective, and botulinum toxin may be used in specific muscle groups for troublesome tremor resistant to other medications. Selegiline and levodopa are used in the treatment of Parkinson's disease and related akinetic–rigid syndromes, and pizotifen as a prophylactic agent in migraine.

175. A: Discontinue the cotrimoxazole

Immune restoration allows discontinuation of prophylaxis for opportunistic infections, provided the CD4 remains at an adequate level. He should remain on three drugs for his HIV. Discontinuing efavirenz will lead rapidly to the development of resistant virus. Despite having an undetectable level of HIV RNA in his blood, it is usually possible to detect virus in the semen, either by RT-PCR, culture or PCR for proviral DNA. He is not allowed by the Department of Health to perform any invasive procedures. BCG is a live vaccine and can cause disseminated disease as he remains immunocompromised.

176. B: Automaticity is mediated by calcium channels

Resting myocytes leak calcium which causes the membrane potential to drift up until an action potential is triggered. The rate of this influx is under autonomic control. Sinus and AV node cells do not have the fast sodium channels responsible for generating action potentials in other myocytes. Potassium efflux restores resting potential. Vagotomy does not abolish automaticity but results in a resting tachycardia.

177. C: It can be administered orally or intravenously

Verapamil is not a dihydropyridine-type calcium-channel blocker (examples of which are nifedipine and nicardipine). The effects of verapamil are mediated by inhibition of slow Ca^{2+} entry to myocardial and conducting tissue, which results in depressant effects on SA and AV node activity. Verapamil is contraindicated in patients with sinoatrial disease, and caution is required when it is combined with β-blockers or digoxin due to potentiation of AV blockade. Oral bioavailability is around 15%, and adverse effects include constipation, nausea and facial flushing. It is useful in suppressing supraventricular arrhythmias, including paroxysmal atrial fibrillation.

178. B: Chi-square test

There are two groups to compare (long versus short course), so A is the least correct (analysis of variance is appropriate when there are more than two groups). Because a single outcome (recurrent attacks) is to be compared between the groups, regression analysis is inappropriate (answer E) and this is the next least correct. The outcome (recurrent attacks, yes/no) is binary and so C and D, which both apply to numeric outcomes, are incorrect. The correct answer is B – the proportions with recurrent attacks could be compared between those given long and short courses of antibiotics using the chi-square test.

179. A: Chest X-ray

Erythema nodosum is a panniculitis typically affecting young women. It may be associated with fever, malaise, arthralgia and arthritis and classically affects the lower limbs. It can be caused by drugs (oral contraceptive pill, penicillins, salicylates, tetracyclines), infections (streptococci, tuberculosis, *Yersinia*, leprosy, psittacosis, and various fungi) and other conditions (inflammatory bowel disease, sarcoidosis, Behçet's disease and malignancy). A chest X-ray must be obtained to exclude sarcoidosis and pulmonary TB.

180. A: Ophthalmoplegia

From this selection, the ophthalmoplegia is the only specific sign of Graves' disease: lid retraction is a non-specific sign of thyrotoxicosis. Clinically, it is difficult to distinguish the diffusely enlarged smooth goitre of Graves' disease from a multinodular goitre, though a goitre with a bruit is diagnostic of Graves' disease.

181. D: Fanconi's anaemia

Fanconi's anaemia is a congenital anaemia with an autosomal recessive pattern of inheritance. The genetic defect is heterogenous.

Patients present with pancytopenia between the ages of five and ten. The disease is associated with growth retardation, skeletal defects, e.g. microcephaly, absent radii or thumbs, renal defects and areas of hyper- and hypopigmentation (*café-au-lait* spots). Cells from patients show an abnormally high frequency of spontaneous chromosomal breakage which is detected in the laboratory by incubating the patient's lymphocytes with diepoxybutane (the DEB test). Ten percent of patients go on to develop acute myeloid leukaemia. Blood counts may improve for a time with androgens but only stem cell transplantation can be curative.

182. E: Sarcoidosis

'Floaters' are suggestive of vitreous inflammation and the reduced vision may be due to macular oedema. Both are features of posterior uveitis and the most common associated systemic disease is sarcoidosis.

183. E: It can be associated with crescentic glomerulonephritis

Exercise-induced haematuria is described in athletes undertaking strenuous physical exercise, such as marathon running or swimming. Renal biopsy is normal in such patients and the haematuria does not reflect underlying glomerular pathology. Here, renal biopsy makes the diagnosis of mesangial IgA disease. IgA disease is the commonest glomerulonephritis worldwide but only 30% of patients progress to end-stage renal failure. It is not associated with hepatitis B infection and typically presents with microscopic haematuria. Only rarely is it a cause of nephrotic syndrome. Any type of glomerulonephritis can undergo acute crescentic change with associated rapid deterioration in renal function.

184. A: Treatment with a combination of a proton pump inhibitor, amoxicillin and clarithromycin

H. pylori is the commonest cause of duodenal ulcer. The positive rapid urease test in this patient confirms *H. pylori* as an aetiological agent. Triple therapy with a combination of proton pump inhibitor and two of the antibiotics (amoxicillin, clarithromycin or metronidazole) is effective in about 90% of cases. Detection of IgG antibody to *H. pylori* is rapid, inexpensive and reliable and so has been widely used for the initial diagnosis. Antibody titres remain elevated for years after successful therapy and are therefore not useful to confirm eradication. Urease breath tests using ^{13}C or ^{14}C are useful to check *H. pylori* eradication and should be performed after discontinuation of proton pump inhibitors to avoid false negatives. Malignant ulcers are very rare in the first part of the duodenum and duodenal ulcers with typical presentation are therefore not routinely biopsied and gastrointestinal endoscopy is not repeated to confirm healing.

185. C: Hearing third person hallucinations discussing her children
The term delusional disorder has replaced paranoid psychosis. It consists of non-bizarre delusions (false, unshakeable beliefs) which persist for at least one month. Tactile (**B**) and olfactory hallucinations can occur as part of the delusion. Auditory hallucinations are uncommon. The third person hallucinations described in the question would be more indicative of paranoid schizophrenia.

186. B: Benefits are dependent on FEV$_1$
Benefits of pulmonary rehabilitation include **decreased** hospitalisations, symptoms, anxiety and depression; and **increased** exercise capacity, quality of life, activities of daily living, and understanding of pulmonary disease, with a possible increase in survival as they are possibly more likely to quit smoking and adhere to mortality-reducing treatments, e.g. long-term oxygen therapy. Benefits are independent of age, FEV$_1$, oxygen dependence, associated disease, and current smoking status.

187. A: Anterior interosseous nerve
This is an anterior interosseous nerve (AIN) palsy; more proximal median nerve or brachial plexus damage is made less likely by the normal sensory examination. The AIN is the largest branch of the median nerve and is motor to flexor pollicis longus, flexor digitorum profundus (thumb and index finger only) and pronator quadratus. It has no cutaneous sensory supply, though it does supply sensory fibres for deep pain and proprioception in several of the wrist joints. Causes of AIN palsy include trauma (rare), external compression (e.g. forearm cast), anomalous fibrous bands in the forearm, or the causes of a mononeuritis.

188. C: Absent HLA-B27 gene
Although plain radiographs are the first line of imaging investigation, they are often insensitive for demonstrating the early changes of sacroiliitis. Although an important feature for establishing the early diagnosis of ankylosing spondylitis (AS), it can only be identified in 50% of cases. Bone scan, CT scan (computed tomography) and, most recently, MRI (magnetic resonance imaging) have been used to

identify sacroiliitis in patients with negative plain sacroiliac radiographs. Using these scan techniques increases the sensitvity for identifying sacroiliitis to 70% of cases. So, a negative plain X-ray (or other scans) does not rule out the diagnosis of AS.

Among whites of Northern European extraction, HLA-B27 occurs in approximately 95% of patients with AS compared with 6% of the general population. Thus, the absence of HLA-B27 indicates that AS is unlikely, unless the patient has classic radiological features. However, absent HLA-B27 does not exclude the possibility of other spondyloarthropathies such as Reiter's syndrome and the arthritis associated with inflammatory bowel disease or psoriasis. In such cases the HLA-B27 is positive in 50–70% of cases. Dual enery X-ray absorptiometry (DEXA) is the gold standard test for the diagnosis and monitoring of osteoporosis, and not AS. However, AS is associated with osteoporosis. A high rate of vertebral fractures occurs with more advanced disease. A small percentage of AS patients have apical pulmonary fibrosis on plain radiographs of the chest. This is mostly asymptomatic and associated with long duration of the disease. It is by no means specific for AS. The ANA is positive in only 10% of patients with AS.

189. C: Noradrenaline (norepinephrine) has greater potency on α receptors than on β receptors

Dobutamine is a relatively selective β_1-agonist, increasing contractility before rate; dopamine acts on dopamine, α and β receptors – it is contentious whether low-dose dopamine has a beneficial affect on renal blood flow independent of its inotropic effect. Noradrenaline acts predominantly on α receptors while adrenaline has more action on β receptors. Aminophylline, a phosphodiesterase inhibitor, prevents breakdown of second messenger cAMP.

190. B: Increased peripheral capillary pressure

Nifedipine is a dihydropyridine calcium-channel blocker that inhibits the slow Ca^{2+} entry phase of depolarisation. Its principal mechanism of action is smooth muscle relaxation, causing vasodilatation, reduced systemic vascular resistance and reduced cardiac afterload. Increased peripheral arterial pressure causes a greater pressure gradient across peripheral capillaries, which predisposes to oedema. Adverse effects of dihydropyridine include enhanced sympathetic activity and activation of the renin-angiotensin system; therefore, a β-blocker or ACE inhibitor can usefully be combined for effective blood pressure lowering. Dihydropyridine, in common with ACE inhibitors and angiotensin-II receptor antagonists, may increase vascular release of nitric oxide, but does not appear to increase sensitivity to nitrates.

191. A: Hypertriglyceridaemia

Loop diuretics act by inhibiting active chloride reabsorption in the ascending limb of the loop of Henle. They can cause a number of metabolic adverse effects, including salt and water depletion, hypochloraemic metabolic alkalosis, hypokalaemia, hypomagnesaemia and hypocalcaemia. Glucose intolerance and reduced urate clearance can also occur, but these are more commonly encountered with thiazide diuretics. Hypertriglyceridaemia has not been described. Deafness can occur following rapid intravenous administration of high doses of loop diuretic.

192. D: Seborrhoeic eczema

Seborrhoeic eczema and seborrhoeic folliculitis are associated with HIV infection, possibly due to an overgrowth of, or abnormal reactivity to *Pityrosporum* yeasts. HIV is also associated with Kaposi's sarcoma and herpes zoster infection, neither of which present in this manner. Kaposi's sarcoma presents with red, brown or purplish macules, nodules or plaques and is associated with human herpesvirus 8 infection. Herpes zoster typically presents with vesiculation.

193. D: Hepatitis C post-exposure prophylaxis (interferon and ribavirin)

Early treatment of acute hepatitis C (HCV RT-PCR-positive, antibody-negative) with interferon and ribavirin appears to have a high success rate, although there are no data on prophylaxis with this combination. Co-amoxiclav is a good broad-spectrum antibiotic for mammalian bites, with Gram-positive, Gram-negative and anaerobic cover. HBV prophylaxis should be given and HIV post-exposure prophylaxis discussed as there has been direct contact with blood.

194. C: Metformin therapy

Metformin treatment is said to be the commonest cause of requests for barium enema examinations from diabetic clinics. The patient has probably not had diabetes long enough to have autonomic neuropathy. Coeliac disease is more common in patients with type 1 diabetes than in the general population (both are 'autoimmune diseases'). To minimise side effects, metformin treatment should be started at a very low dose, increased slowly, and taken regularly as prescribed. The maximum dose may be limited by gastrointestinal side effects.

195. B: Reactive thrombocytosis

This lady's platelet count is raised due to a reactive change because of her iron deficiency. She may be iron deficient because of her obstetric history. She has had two normal deliveries and three first trimester abortions in a six-year period. This is not likely to be due to a haematological cause and is within the limits of normality. Also, her coagulation screen is normal. Causes of a reactive thrombocytosis include haemorrhage, trauma, postoperative, chronic iron deficiency, malignancy, connective tissue diseases, e.g. rheumatoid arthritis, and post-splenectomy.

196. D: Fear she will lose control of herself during an attack

Panic disorder consists of unpredictable episodes of severe anxiety. Physical symptoms occur during panic attacks. Psychological symptoms consist of a fear of dying, going mad or losing control during an attack. Continuous levels of fear are more common in generalised anxiety disorder. A persistent underlying fear of serious disease is indicative of a hypochondriacal disorder. An inability to be reassured that there is no organic illness is indicative of somatisation disorder.

197. B: Aciclovir toxicity

Dialysis dysequilibrium syndrome occurs during the first dialysis in patients who present acutely with markedly elevated urea and creatinine. The history and examination findings do not suggest cerebrovascular accident, which is made unlikely by the normal MRI. Encephalitis, aciclovir toxicity and opiate toxicity are all possibilities. Encephalitis is unlikely to develop three days after starting aciclovir. Haemodialysis patients clear opiates poorly and opiate toxicity will be seen if appropriate dose reductions are not made, even with codeine. However, far more likely in this patient is aciclovir toxicity. Aciclovir is excreted by the kidneys and cleared poorly by dialysis. 400 mg $\times$ 5 per day is a significantly excessive dose and would undoubtedly cause toxicity, which most often manifests as an acute confusional state. An appropriate dose for a dialysis patient would be 400 mg daily.

198. A: Cirrhosis with portal hypertension

The difference between albumin levels in the serum and ascitic fluid, called the serum-ascites albumin gradient (SAAG) is superior to the exudate-transudate concept in the differential diagnosis of ascites. A SAAG of 11 or more is suggestive of ascites associated with portal hypertension. Spontaneous bacterial peritonitis is diagnosed in patients with cirrhosis when the ascitic fluid neutrophil count is more than 250 cells/mm^3. Only 50–80% of these will turn out to have positive ascitic fluid cultures. In patients with cirrhosis and ascites where secondary peritonitis (e.g. perforated viscus, appendicitis) is suspected, a combination of low glucose, high LDH and a very high neutrophil count on the ascitic fluid analysis would strengthen the diagnosis. Ascitic fluid culture under these circumstances would result in the growth of mixed organisms. Pancreatic ascites is characterised by a high ascitic fluid amylase. Demonstration of high triglyceride content in the fluid is essential to distinguish chylous ascites from other causes of a milky white appearance (pseudochylous ascites secondary to cell debris in fluid) of ascitic fluid.

199. E: Optic neuritis

This is a classic presentation of optic neuritis. Unilateral optic nerve compression (e.g. glioma) should be ruled out. Thyroid eye disease is less likely and a pituitary lesion or cavernous sinus thrombosis would result in different symptoms and signs.

Optic neuritis typically presents with the triad of visual loss, abnormal colour vision and eye pain. Of unilateral onset in 70% of patients, it most commonly affects adults in their third decade. Uhthoff's symptom may occur (visual loss worsened by exercise or increase in body temperature – getting in a bath or in hot weather, for example). Visual loss typically occurs over a period of days to reach a peak around 7–10 days, and the majority of patients recover over a few months, sometimes with residual field defects or abnormalities in colour vision or brightness perception.

200. A: Salmeterol has lower lipophilicity

Salmeterol is like salbutamol but has a long N-substituted phenylalkane sidechain attached to a central saligenin nucleus. The saligenin nucleus is responsible for binding to the β_2-adrenoceptor. The long sidechain is responsible for higher lipophilicity; greater bronchial tissue penetration; decreased clearance from the airways; increased resistance to metabolism by catechol-O-methyltransferase; and prolongs binding to a second non-polar domain (**exosite**) on the β_2-adrenoceptor. The effects of salmeterol eventually wear off because of slow dissociation from the exosite and turnover of the occupied β_2-adrenoceptor protein.

201. D: Vasculitis

This patient has asthma, eosinophilia, pulmonary infiltrates, mononeuritis multiplex, and cutaneous lesions. Eosinophilia is associated with various pathological conditions. The patient's presenting features of cough, dyspnoea, and fever could be consistent with chronic eosinophilic pneumonia. Most patients have peripheral eosinophilia, and peripheral infiltrates on chest radiographs. Allergic bronchopulmonary aspergillosis is also characterised by pulmonary infiltrates, commonly with central bronchiectasis. However, our patient's multisystem disease argues against both of these possibilities. Helminthiasis is often accompanied by eosinophilia. During their life cycle, some helminths migrate through the lungs of their hosts, causing transient infiltrates. Pulmonary involvement is a feature of disseminated strongyloidiasis in immunocompromised hosts and has been observed with corticosteroid use. Absence of travel to endemic areas argues against this possibility in our patient. The IHS is characterised by eosinophilia and multi-organ disease, including both pulmonary and neurological findings. Pulmonary involvement in IHS typically includes persistent cough, rather than infiltrates. Cardiac involvement, which was not present in our patient, occurs in about 60% of patients with IHS. Moreover, this diagnosis requires eosinophilia of at least six months' duration. Thus, IHS, although not entirely excluded, seems unlikely. A vasculitic syndrome should be considered most likely. Vessels of any type, in any organ, can be affected, and multi-organ involvement is characteristic of this group of disorders.

202. B: The right coronary artery usually gives rise to the posterior descending artery

The left anterior descending and left circumflex arteries are the main branches of the left main stem artery; the intermediate artery is an occasional variant arising between these. Septal branches arise from the left anterior descending artery, which travels down the anterior interventricular groove. Both sinoatrial and AV nodes are supplied by the right coronary artery in most cases.

203. E: Lisinopril

Digoxin is effective in lowering ventricular rate in atrial fibrillation, and has positive inotropic effects that may improve cardiac output in heart failure. However, digoxin only appears to confer long-term benefits in those heart failure patients with atrial fibrillation, rather than sinus rhythm. Doxazosin is an effective antihypertensive agent that appears to reduce long-term cardiovascular risk, but may be associated with an increased risk of congestive cardiac failure. Loop diuretics and nitrates improve circulating haemodynamics and reduce oedema. However, neither has been shown to reduce the risk of future cardiovascular events or mortality. ACE inhibitors offer a number of advantageous haemodynamic effects (including reduced afterload and improved cardiac output), reduced cardiac remodelling, and reduced progression of atherosclerosis. They have been shown to reduce the occurrence of subsequent myocardial infarction, stroke, and death.

204. D: He has tendon xanthomata

Impaired glucose tolerance and primary hypothyroidism both suggest secondary hyperlipidaemia. Tendon xanthomata are pathognomonic of familial hypercholesterolaemia, while the cholesterol level and family history are non-specific features.

205. C: Acute folic acid deficiency

This patient has been very unwell and ventilated for nine weeks. His illness will increase his folic acid needs. He will be getting total parenteral nutrition but adequate folic acid may not be provided. The patient can then develop an acute deficiency state with macrocytic anaemia, leucopenia and thrombocytopenia. (This is easily missed in ITU because patients are often anaemic, leucopenic and thrombocytopenic for other reasons.) Causes of folic acid deficiency include nutritional (e.g. old age, poverty, special diets, malabsorption (e.g. tropical sprue, coeliac disease), excess utilisation (e.g. pregnancy, prematurity, haemolytic anaemia, myelofibrosis, malignancy and inflammatory disease), drugs which interfere with metabolism (anticonvulsants, sulfasalazine) and mixed (liver disease, alcoholism, intensive care).

206. E: Leptospirosis

Although patients with leptospirosis become jaundiced, frank liver failure is rare. Death usually occurs through renal failure, myocarditis or pulmonary haemorrhage. Renal failure and jaundice (but not conjunctival suffusion) are features of HUS, which has been contracted on campsites where cows have been grazed previously. Brucellosis is not endemic in the UK herd, apart from the very occasional case in an imported animal. Q fever causes a fever, granulomatous hepatitis and pneumonia. Lyme disease does not cause renal failure.

207. D: Aluminium toxicity

Phosphate accumulates in renal failure and is cleared poorly by dialysis. Thus, significant hyperphosphataemia is avoided largely by preventing phosphate absorption from the diet. This is achieved by taking phosphate binders with meals. The commonest phosphate binders are calcium carbonate, calcium acetate and aluminium hydroxide. If taking aluminium hydroxide, plasma aluminium levels must be monitored as accumulation of aluminium causes bone disease, dementia and anaemia. The anaemia of aluminium toxicity is normochromic and normocytic as seen here. Haemolysis in the dialysis circuit is not clinically significant. The patient is receiving a high dose of erythropoietin (EPO) and is iron-replete, making EPO deficiency unlikely. This is not the picture of iron deficiency, with a normal MCV, ferritin and hypochromic red cells. PRCA is an uncommon complication, so far described only with erythropoietin alpha.

208. D: The COX-1 enzyme is involved in mucosal protection

The topical effects of NSAIDs are best described for aspirin. As a weak acid, aspirin is soluble in the low pH of the stomach. It diffuses passively into the mucosa where surface cells are damaged. Local effects of NSAIDs alone are not sufficient to cause significant gastric ulceration and bleeding. Gastropathy in chronic NSAID users is to a major extent a result of systemic prostaglandin inhibition. There are two distinct enzymes that produce prostaglandins. COX-1 is present in most tissues in the body and is responsible for gastric mucosal protection and maintenance of renal blood flow and causes platelet aggregation. COX-2 is produced in response to inflammation. NSAIDs that selectively inhibit COX-2 reduce the risk of gastrointestinal injury. Prostaglandin analogues, such as misoprostol, can reduce the development of gastric and duodenal ulcers. Prophylactic use of H_2-blockers and proton pump inhibitors can reduce the risk of duodenal ulcer in chronic NSAID users.

209. C: Gradual response to high-dose corticosteroids

A patient with acute eosinophilic pneumonia presents with an acute febrile illness of less than five days' duration. They may have severe hypoxaemic respiratory failure requiring ventilation. The chest X-ray shows diffuse infiltrates and bronchoalveolar lavage typically shows a very high (i.e. > 25%) eosinophilia. There is an absence of infection, notably by fungi or parasites. Pulmonary function testing shows a restrictive ventilatory defect (increased FEV_1/FVC ratio, i.e. > 75%) with decreased gas transfer factor (TLCO). High-dose corticosteroids typically result in a quick (within 24 to 48 hours) and complete response that is maintained once they are tapered off.

210. E: He may have osteoporosis and DEXA should be arranged

This man is at risk for osteoporosis and should be evaluated. Baseline DEXA should be performed to assess the patient's fracture risk and, more importantly, to provide a reference point for response to therapy. Although it has been a year since he has taken prednisolone, he had extensive treatment with systemic glucocorticoids prior to this and continues to use high-dose inhaled steroids. Bone loss associated with glucocorticoid therapy occurs in a dose-dependent manner, increasing with greater duration of use and/or magnitude of dose. The threshold for significant risk seems to be oral prednisolone 7.5 mg or more (or equivalent) for six months or longer. Lower doses of prednisolone for extended periods and even prolonged use of inhaled steroids may cause abnormal bone loss. Interestingly, alternate-day dosing of systemic steroids has not been shown to produce less bone loss than daily use.

211. B: First-degree atrioventricular block and left bundle branch block

The three fascicles concerned are the left anterior, left posterior and right. Left anterior hemiblock causes left axis deviation; left posterior hemiblock causes right axis deviation; and right fascicle block causes right bundle branch block. Left bundle branch block requires bifascicular block so a prolonged PR interval is often assumed to represent delay in the right bundle, indicating block in all three fascicles (although the block may in fact be proximal to this). Alternating left and right bundle branch block is also taken to indicate trifascicular disease.

212. C: Nifedipine

Nifedipine has not been proved to reduce mortality in angina patients. Meta-analyses have suggested an increased mortality associated with early short-acting formulations, although combination with a β-blocker appeared to confer benefits above those of β-blockade alone. Newer sustained-release preparations have a smoother pharmacokinetic profile and may be safer. The benefits of aspirin outweigh potential hazards in carefully selected patients; treatment should be avoided in those with low overall cardiovascular risk, uncontrolled hypertension or bleeding diatheses, and should be used with extreme caution if combined with warfarin.

213. A: Squamous cell carcinoma

PUVA therapy consists of UVA with oral 8-methoxypsoralen. It has been shown to predispose to non-melanoma skin cancers (basal and squamous cell carcinoma). There is no increased incidence of seborrhoeic keratoses, pyogenic granuloma or pyoderma gangrenosum with PUVA.

214. B: Oral glucose tolerance test with measurement of growth hormone concentrations

The 'gold standard' for the diagnosis of acromegaly is non-suppression of growth hormone concentrations (and possibly paradoxical elevation) following an oral glucose tolerance test. The normal physiological response is suppression. As growth hormone secretion is pulsatile, a single estimate at any time of day is difficult to interpret. The insulin-like growth factor-1 concentration will be elevated in patients with acromegaly, and is often measured during the diagnostic and treatment phases of their management, but it is not the 'gold standard' diagnostic test.

215. D: Leukaemoid reaction

This very sick and premature baby has a leukaemoid reaction to his infection. Chronic myeloid leukaemia could give a similar raised white cell count but it is excessively rare in a neonate. The bone marrow can increase its cell production in response to stress. This happens particularly easily in neonates. As part of the process there are a lot of nucleated red blood cells (NRBCs) in the peripheral blood. Causes of a neutrophil leucocytosis, which in its extreme form (where there are large numbers of immature circulating white cells) is known as a 'leukaemoid reaction', include bacterial infections, inflammation and tissue necrosis, metabolic disorders, neoplasms, acute haemorrhage or haemolysis, corticosteroid therapy, myeloproliferative disorders and treatment with myeloid growth factors.

216. C: Colour vision should be monitored

Toxicity is very rare with hydroxychloroquine, unlike chloroquine. The most sensitive methods for assessing toxicity are testing of colour vision and corrected reading vision, and assessing for visual distortion using a red Amsler chart. As with chloroquine, patients frequently experience symptoms before any signs are visible. Toxicity is related to the cumulative dose used. Changes are irreversible and may progress on withdrawal of the drug because clearance of hydroxychloroquine from the body is very slow.

217. B: Persistent elevation of mood

The key feature of hypomania is the persistent elevation of mood. This may manifest as elation, but can easily shift to irritability. Energy levels are increased but concentration is often reduced. Mania is more severe than hypomania and can be accompanied by psychotic symptoms, including grandiose delusions and mood-congruent hallucinations.

218. C: Urgent lumbar puncture (LP)

A posterior fossa mass lesion has been ruled out by the normal CT and MRI and the differential diagnosis remains open (e.g. CNS infection, basilar artery thrombosis or other brainstem stroke). His temperature suggests the possibility of CNS infection (although this doesn't rule out the alternative possibility of brainstem stroke) and so an urgent LP, followed by appropriate management depending on the findings, is the best course of action. Steroids are definitely not indicated until the cause of his collapse is established. There is no evidence of subarachnoid haemorrhage to justify treatment with nimodipine, and intravenous heparin is not of established benefit in brainstem stroke.

219. A: Rabies

The incubation periods of tick-borne encephalitis, Japanese encephalitis and West Nile virus infections are less than ten days. HTLV-1 is the cause of tropical spastic paraparesis and does not cause an encephalitis. The incubation of rabies varies from about a week to two years, depending on the site of inoculation and the size of the inoculum.

220. C: Demonstration of C3 nephritic factor would suggest a diagnosis of mesangiocapillary glomerulonephritis

The clinical picture is that of chronic renal failure as demonstrated by small bright kidneys on ultrasound scan. In acute renal failure renal size is normal. The renal failure is most probably due to glomerulonephritis, given the haematuria and proteinuria. Hypertension at presentation is common and, together, the haematuria, proteinuria, hypertension and renal failure constitute the nephritic syndrome. It is not uncommon for renal failure to be diagnosed as an 'incidental' finding when investigating patients for apparently trivial, often unrelated, illnesses. The importance of haematuria and proteinuria must be appreciated. Post-infectious glomerulonephritis causes acute renal failure, not chronic renal failure as seen here. It is most often seen after bacterial, not viral infection. Membranous glomerulonephropathy presents with nephrotic syndrome, not nephritic syndrome. Autosomal dominant polycystic kidney disease (ADPKD) is the only common inherited renal disease to cause renal failure, haematuria and hypertension. It is autosomal dominant, with a 50% chance of offspring inheriting the defect. The ultrasound excludes this diagnosis in this patient. C3 nephritic factor is an autoantibody that stabilises C3 convertase and is seen in mesangiocapillary glomerulonephritis, which typically presents with nephritic syndrome as described here.

221. C: Prothrombin time

Objective and subjective measures are used in the assessment for transplantation in chronic liver disease. The Child-Pugh classification allows objective assessment of patients' functional liver status. Those with grade C cirrhosis have 58%, 21% and 0% one-year, five-year and ten-year survival rates.

Criteria assessed	Points scored for increasing abnormality		
	1	2	3
Encephalopathy	None	1–2	3–4
Ascites	Absent	Mild	Moderate
Serum bilirubin (μmol/l)	<35	35–50	>50
Serum albumin (g/l)	>35	35–28	<28
Prothrombin time prolongation (in seconds)	1–4	4–10	>10
Total score	**<6 A**	**7–9 B**	**>10 C**

Liver enzymes and MCV do not have any impact on the prognosis in patients with cirrhosis.

222. E: Rate of decline of post-bronchodilator FEV$_1$ is significantly decreased

This question involves the ISOLDE trial of FP 500 μg bd versus placebo in COPD patients with a mean FEV$_1$ of 50% predicted. This was a three-year study with 751 subjects. Although the post-bronchodilator FEV$_1$ was higher in the FP group, the **rate of decline** of post-bronchodilator FEV$_1$ was not significantly different between FP and placebo groups. The acute corticosteroid response in this study was assessed with spirometry before and after two weeks of prednisolone 0.6 mg/kg/day.

223. C: Temporal artery biopsy

Jaw claudication is the most specific symptom of giant cell arteritis (GCA). It is easy to elicit when patients describe pain in the jaw area.

However, in many cases the diagnosis is not straightforward. The patient often complains of facial pressure while talking, the reluctance to eat meat because of difficulty in chewing, or inability to open the mouth. The high specificity of jaw claudication is not perfect as it is also encountered in other disorders, such as amyloidosis and atherosclerotic occlusion of the external carotid artery. Therefore, even when the patient tells you that she or he has jaw claudication, a temporal artery biopsy should still be performed to confirm the diagnosis of GCA.

224. D: Multiple blood cultures and observation in hospital pending the result

If a trained operator is present, a transthoracic echo would be useful but the priority in this case is to identify the organism. Multiple blood cultures should be taken from different sites at different times. Transoesophageal echocardiography is required as soon as practical to identify vegetations. Indications for emergency transfer to a tertiary centre include haemodynamic instability (valvular or septic) or evidence of septic embolisation.

225. C: Diltiazem and atenolol

Diltiazem and verapamil are non-dihydropyridine calcium-channel blockers that act predominantly on cardiac conducting tissue to suppress sinoatrial and AV node activity. B-blockers suppress sympathetic cardiac activity and cause delayed AV node conduction. The combination of either verapamil or diltiazem with a β-blocker significantly increases the risk of complete AV node blockade and profound bradycardia, and should generally be avoided or undertaken under specialist supervision.

226. E: Discoid lupus erythematosus

Discoid lupus erythematosus presents in this manner, and is typically aggravated by sunlight. Lesions can cause scarring alopecia. Only a minority of patients progress to systemic symptoms. Gorlin's syndrome is characterised by multiple basal cell carcinomata, palmar pits and jaw cysts; dermatomyositis presents with a heliotropic violaceous discoloration around the eyes; morphoea usually presents with pale indurated plaques which slowly fibrose to cause a slight depression and hyperpigmentation; polymorphic light eruption presents with pruritic erythematous papules in sunlight-exposed sites, but does not present with follicular plugging.

227. E: A dopamine agonist (e.g. bromocriptine or cabergoline)

The first-line treatment for prolactinomas is medical, with dopamine agonists, even for macroadenomas. As well as a biochemical response, the tumour usually shrinks in response to treatment, and pituitary function is preserved. For this reason, it is vital to measure the prolactin concentration preoperatively in any patient with a pituitary tumour.

228. E: All of the above

This patient has a slight lymphocytosis and generalised lymphadenopathy. It is likely that she has a monoclonal lymphoproliferative disorder but a test or tests are needed to prove this in the absence of definitive pathology. Tests which can prove the presence of a monoclonal population are as follows: G6PD and X-linked restriction fragment-length polymorphism (RFLP) analysis in informative females, light-chain restriction in B-lymphoid tumours only, immunoglobulin and *TCR* gene rearrangements in lymphoid malignancies, karyotypic analysis, fluorescent *in situ* hybridisation and detection of a monoclonal population using immunophenotyping by flow cytometry. In the routine clinical setting immunophenotyping would be the first-choice investigation.

229. C: Confusion

Emotional symptoms are common in patients diagnosed with terminal illnesses. Classically, the phases of psychological adjustment to death are denial, anger, bargaining for time, depression and acceptance. Guilt can often occur as part of depression. Anxiety about developing symptoms and a fear of death are also common. Confusion is not common and, if present, the patient should be investigated for possible delirium.

230. B: Acoustic neuroma

These symptoms and signs indicate a cerebellopontine angle lesion, and imply sensorineural deafness on the left. Damage to the left auditory nerve causes Weber's test to lateralise to the opposite (good) side. Together with the gradual onset, this suggests an acoustic neuroma. Acoustic neuroma is one of the most common central nervous system tumours, and there is an association between bilateral acoustic neuromas and neurofibromatosis (type 2). The most consistent early sign of acoustic neuroma is depression or absence of the corneal reflex. Numbness of the face may develop later, though a complete fifth nerve lesion is very unusual. Facial nerve palsy is a late and unusual manifestation (though hemifacial spasm may be a presenting symptom).

231. E: Exhaled carbon monoxide of up to 30 ppm (parts per million) is consistent with smoking abstinence and environmental exposure

Exhaled carbon monoxide is linearly related to blood carboxyhaemoglobin, which has a half-life of approximately four hours. Portable exhaled CO analysers are quick and non-invasive. Exhaled CO levels ≤ 8 ppm suggest recent smoking; 20–30 ppm suggests an average smoker; 80 ppm suggest heavy smoking. Cotinine (a nicotine metabolite) has a half-life of approximately 19 hours and can be easily measured in urine or saliva. Thiocyanates form as a result of hydrogen cyanide in tobacco smoke and can be measured in blood, urine and saliva but can also be formed by eating green vegetables so a dietary history is important.

232. A: Wegener's granulomatosis

In Wegener's granulomatosis (WG), chest radiography may reveal almost any abnormality except hilar adenopathy. Only a few WG patients with hilar adenopathy evident on chest radiographs have been reported. Evidence of hilar adenopathy on a chest radiograph usually places other diseases, particularly sarcoidosis, tuberculosis, and lymphoma, above WG in the differential diagnosis.

233. E: Propylthiouracil

The patient has Graves' thyrotoxicosis (note the thyroid eye disease) and needs treatment for her safety and that of her baby. Radioactive iodine is contraindicated in pregnancy (because of the effect on the fetal thyroid). Operations are best avoided in pregnancy, unless they are essential, though could be done in the second trimester. Of the thionamide drugs, propylthiouracil is probably safer than carbimazole in pregnant and breast-feeding women.

234. C: Staphylococcal toxic shock syndrome

Hyperimmune globulin is used as treatment for tetanus, diphtheria and botulism, and should be given on clinical suspicion alone as the toxin binds irreversibly. Antitoxin is also available for many snake bites, including that of Russell's pit viper. Pooled intravenous immunoglobulin has been used in toxic shock syndrome together with antibiotics, including clindamycin, to inhibit toxin synthesis.

235. A: A urine volume of less than 1 litre/day is a major risk factor for stone formation

In the UK approximately 80% of stones contain calcium. These may range from pure calcium oxalate to a mixture of calcium oxalate and phosphate, to the rare pure calcium phosphate stones. Thus, almost all calcium-containing stones contain calcium oxalate. Only 15–20% of patients who form calcium-containing stones have an underlying disease, the commonest being primary hyperparathyroidism. The most important risk factors for calcium oxalate stone formation are a urinary volume of less than 1 litre/day and hyperoxaluria. Diet contributes significantly to urinary oxalate excretion. Of oxalate excreted in the urine, 85–90% is derived from glyoxylic acid and ascorbic acid metabolism. Oxalate is also absorbed passively in the colon. Calcium in the gut precipitates oxalate, reducing the amount available for absorption. Thus, low dietary calcium is an important determinant of oxalate absorption and therefore urinary oxalate excretion. Hypercalciuria is only important if accompanied by other risk factors. Calcium stone formation is more common in men than in women and 75% of patients who form a stone have a second episode at some time.

236. A: Hospitalisation and intravenous hydrocortisone

This patient has features suggestive of severe acute colitis and the symptoms and sigmoidoscopic features are suggestive of ulcerative colitis (UC) rather than Crohn's disease. 5-aminosalicylates (5-ASAs) are the first-line drugs for mild to moderate UC. Patients with severe colitis (as indicated by six or more, mainly bloody, bowel motions a day, associated constitutional symptoms such as weight loss, pyrexia, tachycardia, anaemia and hypoalbuminaemia) should be hospitalised and treated with intravenous hydrocortisone. Monitoring with plain abdominal X-ray and erect chest X-ray is essential to look for complications such as toxic megacolon and perforation. In patients with severe UC not responding to steroid therapy, intravenous ciclosporin may induce remission. Anti-tumour necrosis factor antibody is indicated in the treatment of refractory, fistulating Crohn's disease.

237. E: Thrombolysis

Pulmonary embolism with hypotension has a grave prognosis if not treated aggressively and ischaemic changes on the ECG is another poor prognostic sign. Pulmonary angiography, which may disperse clot, and surgical embolectomy both carry a high mortality.

Thrombolysis should be undertaken without delay on this patient, there are several regimes with both streptokinase and rt-PA used.

238. B: Streptokinase is a protein produced by group A β-haemolytic streptococci

Fibrinolytic (thrombolytic) drugs break down preformed clot, and are used early in the management of acute myocardial infarction to restore coronary artery patency. Streptokinase causes allergic reactions in around 5% of patients. Administration is associated with development of antibodies, which make subsequent treatments less effective. Therefore, an alternative, such as t-PA, should be used from days 4 to 1 year after streptokinase therapy. Warfarin therapy is not an absolute contraindication to fibrinolytic treatment but the risk of bleeding is increased and caution should be exercised.

239. D: Pyoderma gangrenosum

Pyoderma gangrenosum is an acute inflammatory form of ulceration and is associated with inflammatory bowel disease and rheumatoid arthritis. The rapid history is not typical of the development of a venous ulcer in a patient of this age. Erythema nodosum is associated with inflammatory bowel disease but typically presents with raised tender red nodules. Bowen's disease is squamous cell carcinoma in situ, and presents as a red, scaly lesion. Pyogenic granuloma is a benign, acquired haemangioma which presents as a bright red, raised, sometimes pedunculated lesion which bleeds easily.

240. A: Short Synacthen® test

It is vital not to miss hypocortisolism: a short Synacthen® test may be used to investigate possible secondary hypocortisolism, as the adrenal atrophies without the trophic stimulus of ACTH. Pituitary radiotherapy can continue to have effects for 20 years or more, so it is important to monitor anterior pituitary function long-term. Her dose of thyroxine is unremarkable, making hypothyroidism an unlikely cause of her lethargy. Remember that the TSH is not useful for diagnosing or monitoring the treatment of secondary hypothyroidism: free thyroid hormone concentrations (FT3 or FT4) must be measured. Growth hormone deficiency is a potential cause of her problems, which could be pursued (e.g. by a combination of stems B and C) at leisure.

241. C: Hereditary haemorrhagic telangiectasia

Hereditary haemorrhagic telangiectasia is an autosomal dominant disorder where telangiectasia develop in the skin, mucous membranes and internal organs. They appear in childhood and become more numerous throughout adult life. Patients can have recurrent gastrointestinal haemorrhage and nose bleeding which can lead to chronic iron deficiency. Ten percent of patients have pulmonary arteriovenous malformations. Supportive management includes iron, tranexamic acid, and transfusion if necessary. Treatment of lesions can include embolisation and laser treatment. Oestrogens may increase the severity of blood loss.

242. A: Are normally distributed. Approximately 95% lie within the range (56–84 mmHg)

There is no evidence from the information given that blood pressures were measured inaccurately (E is the least correct). Since the mean and median are approximately equal, this implies that the blood pressures are normally distributed (B and D are therefore incorrect). Approximately 95% will lie within the range mean ± 2 standard deviations (= $70 \pm 2 \times 7 = 56$–84). The approximate 95% confidence interval is given by the mean ± 2 standard ERRORS. Standard error = standard deviation/√sample size = $7/\sqrt{100} = 7/10 = 0.7$ and the approximate 95% confidence interval = $70 \pm 2(0.7) = 68.6$–71.4. D is therefore more incorrect than B, C is incorrect and A is correct.

243. D: Churg-Strauss syndrome

The foot-drop is a clue to the possible presence of mononeuritis multiplex, the causes of which include: diabetes; sarcoidosis; Churg-Strauss; Wegener's granulomatosis; rheumatoid arthritis; SLE; amyloid; carcinoma; polyarteritis nodosa; and leprosy. Respiratory Wegener's granulomatosis (WG) is characterised by dyspnoea, cough, wheeze, haemoptysis, pleurisy and nasal symptoms. Approximately 90% of patients with active WG are cANCA-positive. Consolidation on the Chest X-ray is uncommon in WG and one would more usually expect to find nodules that cavitate. Kartagener syndrome is associated with sinusitis and bronchiectasis but pulmonary shadowing is not classically flitting in nature. ABPA could fit the respiratory features but the foot-drop does not fit in. Churg-Strauss syndrome has all the features listed above and is associated with a positive ANCA in only approximately 50% cases. It is therefore the best answer that ties all the features together.

244. C: Dermatomyositis (DM)

This patient presented with proximal muscle weakness and significantly raised muscle enzymes. The possible diagnoses include inflammatory myopathy and muscular dystrophy. The distinctive rash over the knuckles (Grotton rash), elbows, and eyelids (heliotrope rash) is typical of DM. It can occur at any age. It is more common in women than men. Myositis changes on EMG (short-duration, polyphasic motor unit potentials with spontaneous fibrillation potentials) and muscle biopsy are often used to confirm the diagnosis.

245. B: Centrocaecal scotoma

Toxic amblyopia is typically bilateral and most often seen in patients who use alcohol or tobacco excessively; malnutrition (e.g. vitamin B_{12} deficiency) may coexist. Visual disturbance develops insidiously over weeks to months, with enlarging central or pericentral scotomata. When the scotoma involves both the fovea (fixation) and the blind spot it is known as a 'centrocaecal scotoma'. Disc pallor is associated with toxic amblyopia but may also reflect coexistent vitamin B_{12} deficiency. Homonymous hemianopia is most often seen with contralateral lesions of the occipital cortex (e.g. stroke); bi-temporal hemianopia with optic chiasm lesions; and altitudinal field defects with ischaemic optic nerve lesions.

246. C: Haemorrhagic smallpox

All of the infections listed, including smallpox, can give this clinical picture. Smallpox is the least likely as it no longer exists in the wild. *Capnocytophaga canimorsus* (formerly known as 'DF-2') is acquired from dog bites and causes a particularly severe infection in splenectomised patients.

247. B: Secondary hyperparathyroidism is treated with the 1-alpha-hydroxylated form of vitamin D

This patient has hypercalcaemia in the setting of a normal, not suppressed, PTH. The diagnosis is therefore tertiary hyper-parathyroidism. In secondary hyperparathyroidism the calcium is low, driving appropriate 'physiological' PTH production. Hypercalcaemia of inflammatory conditions responds to corticosteroids. The kidney undertakes 1-alpha-hydroxylation of cholecalciferol and the liver, 25-hydroxylation. 1,25 dihydroxy-cholecalciferol both ensures normal calcification of bone and directly inhibits PTH release. Thus, in renal failure 1-alpha-hydroxylated vitamin D_3 is given in order to prevent development of tertiary hyperparathyroidism and renal osteodystrophy. Tertiary hyperparathyroidism may be controlled with appropriate medical management, not always requiring parathyroidectomy. Transplantation replaces endogenous 1-alpha-hydroxylation, restoring normal calcium phosphate balance in most patients.

248. D: Roth spots

Extracardiac manifestations of bacterial endocarditis include: conjunctival haemorrhages, Roth spots, splinter haemorrhages, Osler's nodes, Janeway lesions, splenomegaly, renal complications and cerebral vasculitis.

Roth spots are retinal haemorrhages with a pale centre result from small vessel vasculitis. Silver- or copper wiring is a description of increased reflectivity of retinal vessels regarded by physicians as the result of hypertension (grade 1 hypertensive retinopathy) but disputed by many ophthalmologists, who regard this as normal. Hard exudates are most frequently seen in diabetic retinopathy. There are many causes of the appearance of papilloedema, which can broadly be divided into raised pressure and inflammation. Optic atrophy is the result of degeneration of the disc and may be the end result of inflammation, mechanical stress, ischaemia or primary degeneration.

249. D: Type 1 aortic dissection

An aortic dissection has occurred involving the ostium of the right coronary and causing a pericardial tamponade. Kawasaki disease can cause infarction and pericardial effusion but generally occurs in infants. A massive pulmonary embolism or posterior myocardial infarction could cause the chest pain, hypotension, tachycardia and some ECG changes but not an immediate pericardial effusion. Viral pericarditis may cause all the signs but presents less acutely.

250. C: Correction of fluid and electrolyte abnormalities

Digoxin toxicity is enhanced by volume depletion, hypokalaemia, hypercalcaemia, and hypomagnesaemia. After discontinuing digoxin treatment, management is generally supportive and includes careful attention to fluid and electrolyte balance. Loop diuretics are likely to worsen the features of digoxin toxicity. Lidocaine (lignocaine) or phenytoin may be effective where digoxin-induced ventricular tachyarrhythmias occur. Calcium gluconate may be a useful adjunct in hyperkalaemia but has no proved role in digoxin toxicity. Specific F_{AB} antibody fragments enhance drug clearance, and may be of value in life-threatening digoxin toxicity. Dialysis may enhance drug clearance, but has not been proved to be of clinical value.

251. B: Start him on an ACE inhibitor (ACEI)

The patient has microalbuminuria: the use of an ACEI will slow the progression of his diabetic nephropathy. His blood pressure target should be less than 120/70 mmHg. Given his normal creatinine, a renal ultrasound scan is not indicated. A urinary tract infection would be likely to cause dipstick proteinuria rather than microalbuminuria. He has no haematuria, and the other features of his case do not indicate a need to pursue other causes of renal dysfunction.

252. A: Sickle cell anaemia

This boy has anaemia with reticulocytosis, raised bilirubin and LDH, suggesting haemolysis. He has symptoms and signs of dactylitis caused by infarcts of the small bones. This will not lead to X-ray changes immediately although later in life it may lead to marked shortening of bones. All of these features support a diagnosis of sickle cell anaemia. He is of Ghanaian origin, a high-incidence area, and was born in a very low-incidence area for haemoglobinopathy where routine neonatal screening will not be offered. Sickle cell anaemia is due to a point mutation on the β-globin gene. Hb SS is insoluble and forms crystals in low oxygen tensions. Deoxygenated sickle haemoglobin polymerises, leading to sickling of red cells, which block the microcirculation or large vessels. Clinically, this leads to painful vaso-occlusive crises (in bones, lungs, spleen and brain), visceral sequestration crises, aplastic crises and haemolytic crises.

253. A: Paraneoplastic syndrome

Paraneoplastic syndromes may present with ataxia, subacute confusion, oculomotor disorders, visual loss or a peripheral neuropathy. This presentation, with peripheral neuropathy-like signs, ataxia and a cerebellar syndrome would be compatible with a paraneoplastic disorder. Cerebellar degeneration is associated with lung cancer and the anti-Yo autoantibody (to Purkinje cells in the cerebellum). The case history described could also potentially be an unusual presentation of Creutzfeldt-Jakob disease.

254. B: Is associated with organising pneumonia

ILD in polymyositis is more common with a normal CK and is independent of myositis severity. ILD may occur before or after the development of polymyositis. A number of pulmonary histological appearances can result, including fibrosing alveolitis, organising pneumonia, and diffuse alveolar damage. TLCO is decreased in both ILD and respiratory muscle weakness, although in pure respiratory muscle weakness there may be a supranormal gas transfer coefficient (KCO). Fibrosing alveolitis in polymyositis is associated with the presence of t-RNA synthetases (autoantibodies directed against soluble cellular antigens), e.g. anti-Jo-1 and anti-PL-12. Treatment consists of systemic corticosteroids with/without immunosuppressants such as azathioprine and cyclophosphamide.

255. E: Norovirus

Norovirus (also known as Norwalk virus and SRSV) has recently spread in many UK hospitals, necessitating the closure of wards as patients and staff have developed the disease. Enteroviruses hardly ever cause gastrointestinal symptoms, but cause conditions such as aseptic meningitis, encephalitis, hand, foot and mouth disease, myocarditis, and Bornholm disease.

256. A: Aspirate the synovial fluid from the left knee

Acute pain and swelling in a joint always require immediate evaluation, even if the patient is known to have established chronic arthritis in that joint. Although there are many other less life-threatening causes of monoarthritis, inadequately treated infectious arthritis carries a risk of prolonged morbidity and even mortality. If untreated, some infections can destroy cartilage in as little as one to two days. High-risk groups include the immunocompromised, individuals who use intravenous drugs, and those with an underlying arthritis (especially patients with rheumatoid arthritis). Patients with rheumatoid arthritis have two to three times the mortality of non-rheumatoid patients and early diagnosis and treatment in these individuals is imperative. Any patient with rheumatoid arthritis who comes in with symptoms/signs in one joint out of proportion to disease activity elsewhere should have that joint aspirated and a fluid sample sent urgently for Gram stain and culture and sensitivity.

257. D: β-Blocker, ACE inhibitor, spironolactone

Of all the options this is unequivocally the best, although spironolactone is the most contentious of the three. Clearly the patient should also be on some form of antiplatelet or anticoagulant treatment. Adding angiotensin-II blockers to a regime including β-blockers and ACE inhibitors may actually worsen prognosis although they should be prescribed where ACE inhibitors are not tolerated.

258. A: Acute tubular necrosis

The patient is intravascularly volume-depleted with a postural drop in blood pressure. She has a mild pyrexia and a tachycardia. Pyelonephritis is an uncommon complication of urinary tract infection. The absence of tachycardia and abdominal tenderness argue against this diagnosis. Interstitial nephritis is unlikely to present 24 hours after starting ciprofloxacin. No history or investigations to support a diagnosis of haemolytic uraemic syndrome (HUS) are given. Post-infectious glomerulonephritis complicates bacterial upper respiratory tract infection not urinary tract infection. A patient with diabetic nephropathy is at increased risk of acute tubular necrosis in the setting of significant intravascular volume depletion.

259. C: Co-amoxiclav

The biochemical pattern presented is indicative of cholestatic jaundice. This can occur during or shortly after administration of co-amoxiclav, and is more likely in elderly patients. Nitrofurantoin is effective in treating lower urinary tract infection; cholestatic jaundice has been reported, but occurs rarely. Flucloxacillin can cause cholestatic jaundice, but is inappropriate treatment for a lower urinary tract infection and unlikely to have been used in this setting. It is active against *Staphylococcus aureus*, and is used to treat cellulitis, osteomyelitis, and aspiration pneumonia.

260. D: Hypocalcaemia is related to fat malabsorption

The classic triad of pancreatic calcification, steatorrhoea, and diabetes mellitus establishes the diagnosis of chronic pancreatitis, but is found in less than one-third of the patients. When a plain X-ray is negative, computed tomography of the abdomen or endoscopic ultrasound may demonstrate parenchymal and ductal abnormalities. Endoscopic retrograde cholangiopancreatography should preferably be reserved for those for whom therapeutic intervention is intended.

Faecal fat concentration of $\geq$ 9.5% is typical of steatorrhoea. Vitamin D is a fat-soluble vitamin and hypocalcaemia could result, secondary to vitamin D deficiency. D-xylose urinary excretion is a test for carbohydrate absorption, which is usually normal in these cases because patients with defective intraluminal digestion usually absorb xylose normally as long as the mucosal structure is normal. The bentiromide test uses synthetic peptide benzoyl-tyrosyl-p-aminobenzoic acid (BT-PABA), which is cleaved by chymotrypsin, liberating PABA. The PABA metabolite excreted in the urine is measured to assess pancreatic exocrine function. Cobalamin (vitamin B_{12}) malabsorption can occur in 40% of patients with alcoholic chronic pancreatitis and in most patients with cystic fibrosis. This may be due to excessive binding of B_{12} to the non-intrinsic factor cobalamin-binding protein. The latter is usually destroyed by pancreatic proteases. In pancreatic insufficiency the protein competes with intrinsic factor, resulting in B_{12} malabsorption.

261. C: Prevention of ischaemic heart disease

Recent evidence from prospective randomised placebo-controlled studies (Heart and Estrogen/progestin Replacement Study II (HERS II) and the Women's Health Initiative Study (WHI)), has not shown any evidence that HRT prevents ischaemic heart disease. This contradicts the results of previous observational studies. Prevention of ischaemic heart disease or stroke is no longer an indication for the prescription of HRT. HRT may be used to treat menopausal symptoms, and to prevent osteoporosis (though the targeted use of more effective anti-osteoporotic agents may be preferred). The individual risk/benefit profile needs to be considered for each patient.

262. E: Common peroneal nerve

The common peroneal nerve can be damaged by trauma where it wraps around the head of the fibula. It is motor to the peronei and tibialis anterior muscles, so damage causes foot-drop. A common peroneal nerve lesion can be distinguished from an L5 root lesion by the presence of weak foot inversion and eversion in the former. In addition, the nerve is sensory to a small patch on the dorsum of the foot near the web space between the big and second toes, although a common peroneal nerve lesion often presents with little or no sensory loss. In addition to traumatic lesions, diabetes, polyarteritis and the other causes of mononeuritis must be excluded.

263. C: Stage IIIB

The disease is at stage IIIB as the patient has lymph nodes above and below the diaphragm and symptoms of night sweats and weight loss. Stage I indicates involvement of one lymph node area. Stage II indicates disease of two more lymph nodal areas on the same side of the diaphragm. Stage III indicates disease involving disease above and below the diaphragm. Splenic disease is included in stage III but has special significance. Stage IV indicates involvement outside the lymph node areas and refers to diffuse or disseminated disease in the bone marrow, liver and other extranodal sites. The stage number is followed in all cases by the letter A or B indicating the absence (A) or presence (B) of one or more of the following: unexplained fever above 38 °C, night sweats, loss of more than 10% of body weight in the last six months. As involvement of the spleen is often a prelude to widespread haematogenous spread, patients with lymph node involvement and splenic involvement are staged as III.

264. A: Chickenpox

Primary varicella in early pregnancy leads to infection of the fetus which then develops episodes of shingles-like attacks. If these occur over a developing limb bud or in the trigeminal distribution, that area fails to develop properly over the ensuing weeks. If it occurs over the trunk, a scar develops. The incidence of attributable fetopathy is probably about 2%. Secondary syphilis and CMV do not cause focal developmental problems. Parvovirus B19 infection may result in either miscarriage or hydrops fetalis (oedema caused by fetal cardiac failure, due to anaemia caused by viral infection of fetal erythroblasts). Rubella vaccine is a live attenuated vaccine. It infects the fetus but has never been associated with any damage to the fetus (and has been given to many women who did not realise they were pregnant at the time).

265. D: Carbon monoxide poisoning

The clue to the diagnosis of CO poisoning is the discrepancy between SaO_2 and PaO_2. Most pulse oximeters use only two light wavelengths to measure the oxy-/deoxyhaemoglobin ratio. However, at the shorter wavelength (660 nm), carboxyhaemoglobin and oxyhaemoglobin have similar absorption of light and this tricks the oximeter into thinking it is measuring oxyhaemoglobin when it is actually measuring carboxyhaemoglobin. This can be overcome by using a CO-oximeter, which uses at least four light wavelengths and differentiates better between carboxyhaemoglobin and oxyhaemoglobin. Once confusion is a feature then carboxyhaemoglobin level is at 40–60% and the patient is at risk of respiratory failure and death.

266. E: Osteopetrosis

Osteopetrosis is a rare disease of greatly increased bone density (marble bone disease). It results from defective osteoclast function with a failure of normal bone resorption. Paget's disease may affect one or many bones, but in the majority of patients most of the skeleton is uninvolved. The pathology is characterised by a mixed osteolytic and osteoblastic mosaic. Osteoporosis is defined pathologically as an absolute decrease in the amount of bone, leading to fractures after minimal trauma. Osteogenesis imperfecta (OI) is a heritable defect in type I collagen synthesis that results primarily in fragile bones that break with minimal trauma. Osteomalacia is defined as an increase in the osteoid seam width, accompanied by a decrease in the mineralisation front.

267. E: Pneumothorax

Haemodialysis machines have bubble traps and alarms to detect air in the dialysis circuit, making air embolism extremely unlikely. However, if it occurs hypotension results. Dysequilibrium is seen in patients such as this, presenting acutely, as a result of the large shifts in metabolites when dialysis is first given. It is effectively prevented by phenytoin. The weight loss for this patient is modest. This and the blood pressure post-dialysis exclude excessive fluid removal and resulting intravascular volume depletion. Pericardial tamponade would also be associated with hypotension. The most likely diagnosis is pneumothorax secondary to central line insertion. A chest X-ray should always be performed after line insertion but is not commented on here, possibly as the patient is acutely unwell with a markedly elevated urea and it was decided that it was necessary to proceed to dialysis without delay.

268. B: He could transmit hepatitis B to his partner if he is hepatitis Be antigen-positive

Hepatitis B is a DNA virus that is transmitted parenterally, vertically as well as through sexual contacts. Intact virion consists of an outer coat and an inner core. The serological test to detect the virus identifies hepatitis B surface antigen (HBsAg). The antigen expressed on the nucleocapsid core is the hepatitis B core antigen (HBcAg), which does not circulate in the serum. A third antigen, hepatitis Be antigen (HBeAg) is a degradation product of pre-core protein and indicates infectivity. Laboratory diagnosis of hepatitis B infection is based on the detection of different antigens and antibodies in the serum, the level of liver enzymes, and the detection of viral DNA in the serum and necro-inflammation in liver biopsy. Liver biopsy is not indicated if viral DNA is not detectable and liver enzymes are normal on three occasions. The following patterns of test results are seen in clinical practice:

Acute infection: HBsAg+, anti-HBc+ (IgM)
Resolved infection: HBsAg–, anti-HBc+ (IgG)
Hep. B vaccination: HBsAg–, Anti-HBs+

Inactive carrier: HBsAg+ > 6 months
   HBeAg–, anti-HBe+
   HBV DNA <10^5 copies/ml
   Normal liver enzymes
Chronic hepatitis: HBsAg+ > 6 months
   HBeAg+/–
   HBV DNA >10^5 copies/ml
   Raised liver enzymes
   Necro-inflammation on liver biopsy

269. E: Restrictive myocardial disease

The osteopenia, anaemia, raised ESR and globulins, and proteinuria all point to myeloma. Myeloma is associated with AL amyloid which may cause infiltration of myocardium and a restrictive picture. Clinically, this can be extremely hard to differentiate from constriction but where an aetiological disease coexists this should be treated as prime suspect. Other causes of restrictive myocardial disease include sarcoidosis, endomyocardial fibrosis and connective tissue disease.

270. E: Nebulised salbutamol

The initial management of acute asthma involves administration of oxygen, salbutamol (nebulised in oxygen), and intravenous hydrocortisone (e.g. 200 mg). Salbutamol is most likely to improve her immediate condition; nebulised formulations have greater effectiveness than metered-dose inhalers because of the smaller particulate size, and better delivery to the site of action. Intravenous hydrocortisone is administered early to reduce respiratory mucosal oedema and inflammation. However, clinical benefit is not obtained until several hours after administration. Ipratropium bromide (anticholinergic) may offer some improvement in combination with salbutamol, but is significantly less effective than salbutamol as monotherapy; it is thought to have greater efficacy in chronic obstructive pulmonary disease. Aminophylline is reserved for patients who fail to respond adequately to oxygen, salbutamol and hydrocortisone. Intravenous antibiotics may be required if clinical signs or investigations suggest infection, but is unlikely to offer any immediate benefits.

271. A: Vertebral artery dissection

Besides trauma (which can be trivial, as this case illustrates), various causes of vertebral artery dissection have been reported, including hypertension, drug abuse, migraine, and cervical manipulation. The result of the arterial dissection is a sudden intrusion of blood into the arterial wall which results in the creation of a false lumen that may occlude the vessel or propagate thrombus. Patients with vertebral artery dissection may present with minor symptoms such as headache and neck pain, but severe and catastrophic neurological deficits occur if crucial branch vessels become occluded. For example, the posterior inferior cerebellar artery (PICA) territory can be infarcted, affecting not only the posterior inferior cerebellum, the cerebellar tonsils and ipsilateral vermis, but also the dorsolateral portion of the medulla. This is known as Wallenberg's syndrome (see question 113).

272. C: Chronic hepatitis C

He has cryoglobulinaemia secondary to chronic HCV infection. HIV-associated nephropathy is a focal segmental glomerulosclerosis. HBV is associated with a membranoproliferative glomerulonephritis, but not the rash of cryoglobulinaemia. *Staphylococcus aureus* endocarditis commonly causes a vasculitic rash, but the illness is usually more rapidly progressive. It produces a mesangioproliferative glomerulonephritis. Post-streptococcal glomerulonephritis is a diffuse proliferative glomerulonephritis.

273. A: Acute gout is a recognised adverse effect

Allopurinol is a prodrug that is converted to oxypurinol and acts as a xanthine oxidase inhibitor to reduce urate production from purine metabolism. It inhibits hepatic enzyme activity, which can reduce the metabolism of warfarin, thereby increasing the risk of bleeding. Allopurinol is indicated for gout prophylaxis, urate nephropathy (including tumour lysis syndrome), asymptomatic hyperuricaemia, and asymptomatic hyperuricuria. Initiation of urate-lowering therapy can provoke acute gout, which may require treatment with a non-steroidal anti-inflammatory drug (NSAID) or colchicine. Allopurinol may be safely combined with a NSAID. However, allopurinol combined with azathioprine or 6-mercaptopurine is potentially hazardous because the latter two drugs are usually metabolised by xanthine oxidase and the risks of bone marrow toxicity are increased.

274. A: Alendronate

From this list, the bisphosphonates have the best data for the prevention of osteoporotic fractures. Etidronate can predispose to the development of osteomalacia, which is not a problem with the newer, more effective bisphosphonates (e.g. alendronate, risedronate). You should also be aware of raloxifene as another evidence-based way to prevent osteoporosis. Raloxifene is a selective oestrogen receptor modulator (SERM) with oestrogen-agonist effects in some tissues (e.g. bone) and oestrogen-antagonist effects in others (e.g. breast).

275. **B: The scar is likely to have formed before the age of ten years**
The radiological investigations make the diagnosis of reflux nephropathy. As with many chronic renal disease, reflux nephropathy may be undetected until routine investigations reveal proteinuria, renal impairment or hypertension. Pregnancy is one such occasion. Furthermore, glomerular hyperfiltration is seen normally in pregnancy. In patients with underlying renal disease, such as reflux nephropathy, this may precipitate hypertension, proteinuria and deterioration in excretory renal function. The radiological appearances are diagnostic, biopsy not being necessary. Reflux of infected urine is believed to be essential in the pathogenesis of reflux nephropathy. As with most chronic renal disease, the presence of proteinuria is a marker for subsequent progressive renal failure.

276. **D: Serology for *E. histolytica* is positive in > 90% of cases**
E. histolytica causes ulceration in the terminal ileum and right colon, although the rest of the colon can also be involved. Symptoms range from a few foul-smelling loose motions to a fulminant attack presenting with dysentery and systemic symptoms. Protozoa invade the portal circulation to reach the liver and cause liver abscesses. There is often an interval of a few months between the manifestation of bowel symptoms and the presentation with liver abscess. Concurrent bowel symptoms are therefore rare in those presenting with liver abscess. A history of dysentery is elicited in less than one-half of the patients with liver abscess. Yield from stool examination is low in those with liver abscess, with only one-third of cases demonstrating trophozoites or cysts. Ultrasound (abdomen) would demonstrate one or more hypoechoic lesions within the liver, typical of an abscess. Serological tests are positive in over 90% of these cases. Liver enzymes show varying degrees of change, with marked elevation of alanine transaminase and jaundice indicating a poor prognosis. Treatment with a tissue amoebicide, such as metronidazole, should be followed by a course of luminal amoebicide, such as diloxanide furoate, to eradicate the trophozoites dwelling in the bowel lumen. Radiological or surgical drainage is only indicated in cases where there is impending rupture or intense pain due to a tense abscess which does not resolve on

medical treatment. Pus from the abscess consists mainly of necrotic liver tissue and neutrophils, and *E. histolytica* are not usually seen on microscopy.

277. C: Can be administered as an inhaled powder or aerosol or nebulised solution

Disodium cromoglicate is used in the prophylaxis of asthma; it is ineffective in the treatment of acute attacks. It can precipitate acute bronchospasm, especially when inhaled in powder form, but this can be avoided by concomitant administration of inhaled salbutamol. Its mechanism of action is unclear, but it is believed to act by stabilising mast cells and preventing degranulation and release of bronchoconstricting factors (e.g. histamine and prostaglandins). It appears to be more effective in younger patients, and can effectively prevent exercise-induced asthma.

278. D: Acquired haemophilia

Acquired haemophilia is due to the development of an inhibitor to factor VIII in a non-haemophiliac. The antibody is usually IgG. The inhibitors develop in the elderly, in pregnancy and the puerperium, and in association with autoimmune disorders, malignancy, various skin disorders, infections and drug therapy. The patients present with bleeding (e.g. postoperatively) and bruising. Haemarthrosis is rare. There is a significant associated mortality. Laboratory investigation demonstrates a prolonged APTT, decreased factor VIII level and the presence of antibody to factor VIII with a specific antibody assay. Treatment involves immune suppression of the antibody using steroids and cyclophosphamide.

279. A: Dyspnoea

According to the Prospective Investigation of Pulmonary Embolism Diagnosis (PIOPED) data, in order of frequency, the commonest symptoms in women with PE are: dyspnoea (80%); pleuritic chest pain (60%); cough (41%); leg swelling (24%); and haemoptysis (10%). The figures for men are 78%, 57%, 40%, 36% and 21% respectively.

280. C: Pyoderma gangrenosum

Pyoderma gangrenosum is deep, red, necrotic ulcers with undermined, violaceous, oedematous borders. These lesions typically evolve over the lower limbs. The ulcers have ragged bluish-red overhanging edges and a necrotic base. While pyoderma gangrenosum may be an isolated finding it is most often associated with other disorders such as inflammatory bowel disease, RA and Wegener's granulomatosis. Fixed drug eruptions (FDEs) characteristically recur in the same site or sites each time a particular drug is taken. The typical cutaneous reaction consists of round or oval patches of redness and swelling of the skin, sometimes surmounted by a blister. Sulphonamides, non-steroidal anti-inflammatory drugs and tetracyclines are frequently implicated. This patient is on a sulphonamide-containing drug but the lesions in the legs are ulcerative and not typical of FDEs. Although rheumatoid nodules may ulcerate and get infected, the location of the ulcers on the anterior part of the leg is not typical for rheumatoid nodules. Vasculitic skin rash is a plausible alternative diagnosis in this case, although, the necrotic skin lesions are often smaller and have no overhanging edge. RA is associated with erythema nodosum in 3–5% of cases. It presents with characteristic painful, red skin nodules, usually on the front of the legs. They vary in size between a cherry and a grapefruit, and in number from two to fifty or more. They rarely ulcerate.

281. **E: Mycophenolate mofetil acts more selectively on lymphocytes**
Stimulation of T-cell receptors results in calcineurin activation, a process inhibited by ciclosporin and tacrolimus. Calcineurin dephosphorylates nuclear factor of activated T cells (NFAT), enabling the latter to enter the nucleus and bind to interleukin-2 (IL-2) promoter. Corticosteroids act on cytosolic receptors, inhibiting cytokine gene transcription in lymphocytes and antigen-presenting cells. IL-2-receptor stimulation induces cells to proliferate. This could be inhibited by IL-2-receptor antibodies or by sirolimus (Rapamune®), which inhibits second-messenger signals induced by IL-2. Azathioprine and mycophenolate mofetil (MMF) interrupt DNA replication by inhibiting purine synthesis. MMF inhibits inosine monophosphate, blocking the *de novo* pathway of purine synthesis selective to lymphocytes. Ciclosporin stimulates TGF-β production, which is responsible for the chronic nephrotoxic side effects of ciclosporin. Tacrolimus antagonises TGF-β and is associated with less hirsutism and gum hypertrophy, but up to 20% of patients develop diabetes mellitus. MMF is associated with diarrhoea.

282. **D: Brown-Séquard syndrome**
Brown-Séquard syndrome is characterised by a clinical picture reflecting hemisection of the spinal cord, often in the cervical cord

region. It is usually incomplete. The signs reflect spinal cord anatomy:

1. Interruption of the lateral corticospinal tracts causing ipsilateral pyramidal (upper motor neurone) weakness below the level of the lesion, and an ipsilateral extensor plantar.
2. Interruption of the dorsal (posterior) columns which carry ipsilateral vibration and joint-position sense. These senses are therefore lost ipsilaterally below the level of the lesion.
3. Interruption of the lateral spinothalamic tracts, causing contralateral loss of pain and temperature sensation. This usually occurs two to three segments below the level of the lesion.

The progressive nature of the disorder makes a lumbosacral disc prolapse or vascular cause (spinal artery occlusion) less likely and the symptoms are not typical for Guillain-Barré syndrome or syringomyelia.

283. B: Left atrial myxoma

The mitral stenosis-like murmur is caused by the tumour prolapsing through the mitral valve – this is positional, hence the odd but severe orthopnoea. Infective endocarditis causes regurgitant murmurs; sinus of Valsalva aneurysms are a late complication of endocarditis and can rupture into the right ventricle causing an AV shunt.

284. B: Amoebic liver abscess

Typically, amoebic abscesses occur in the right lobe of the liver and are single abscesses without septa. They are associated with a neutrophilia and respond well to metronidazole. Aspiration is indicated if the abscess is about to rupture or for diagnosis if there is a probability that the abscess is bacterial. Diagnosis of amoebic abscesses is by serology. Amoebic liver abscess is a common problem in the developing world and is particularly common in Mexico City. Cysticercosis cysts are small (1 cm) and are not associated with an acute febrile illness. Hydatid cysts can be large, but are usually multiple or septate and are not associated with fever unless they become infected. Hepatic actinomycosis follows a much slower course.

285. A: Allopurinol

Carbemazepine, griseofulvin, phenytoin and rifampicin are all hepatic enzyme inducers that increase metabolism of the COCP and thereby reduce its circulating concentrations and effectiveness.

It should be remembered that cigarette smoking also induces hepatic enzymes and may have a clinically significant effect on COCP metabolism in certain individuals. Allopurinol is a xanthine oxidase inhibitor which can inhibit hepatic enzyme activity.

286. D: A venous bicarbonate concentration of 8 mmol/l

Patients with newly diagnosed type 2 diabetes are 'allowed' one plus (and possibly two pluses) of ketonuria on dipstick urinalysis. There may well be some weight loss in the period immediately prior to their diagnosis. Although there is often a family history of type 2 diabetes, this is not necessarily the case. Patients often have multiple features of the metabolic syndrome X, including hypertension, but not all patients with type 2 diabetes are hypertensive. The finding of a low venous bicarbonate is suggestive of insulin deficiency, and the most worrying of the features the GP has described.

287. C: Focal segmental glomerulosclerosis

The history is typical of HIV-associated nephropathy (HIVAN). Presentation is most often with heavy proteinuria in the setting of mild impairment of excretory renal function and normal blood pressure. It may occur in any HIV-positive patient and is not restricted to intravenous drug abusers as originally believed. It is ten times more common in black African and African-American patients than in white patients. More than 50% of patients with nephrotic syndrome due to HIVAN are asymptomatic, seropositive HIV carriers or have AIDS-related complex (ARC). Ultrasound scan reveals large echogenic kidneys in the nephrotic stage of the illness and focal segmental glomerulosclerosis is seen on biopsy in approximately 80% of cases. Classically, a rapid progression to end-stage renal failure is seen.

288. B: Hepatocellular carcinoma needs to be excluded

Serology suggests past resolved hepatitis B infection, so it is likely that this patient is likely to have hepatitis C-related cirrhosis. In the UK 0.5–1% of the population are infected with hepatitis C virus. Of those infected, 85% develop chronic hepatitis. Although the rate of progression varies among different populations, about 20% develop cirrhosis over a 20-year period, of whom 30% develop hepatocellular carcinoma over 30 years of follow-up. Higher age at infection, male gender, infection acquired by blood products, associated HIV or HBV infection and alcohol excess predict increased rates of progression. Chronic hepatitis C is treated with a combination of polyethylene glycolated (PEG) interferon and ribavirin for 6 to 12 months. Genotypes 1 and 4 are more resistant to antiviral therapy than genotypes 2 and 3. Sustained response is seen in about 55% treated with the combination therapy. Patients with decompensated cirrhosis do not tolerate antiviral therapy well. Hepatitis C invariably recurs after liver transplantation and up to 25% go on to develop cirrhosis of the transplanted liver.

289. C: Co-careldopa

Parkinson's disease is characterised by a relative deficiency of dopamine (DA) in the substantia nigra cells of the basal ganglia, resulting in extrapyramidal clinical features. Levodopa is converted to DA by the enzyme dopa decarboxylase. Inhibition of dopa decarboxylase in the peripheral circulation allows greater concentrations of levodopa to cross the blood–brain barrier; this increases efficacy, and reduces peripheral DA-induced adverse effects (nausea, hypotension). Therefore, levodopa is usually combined with benserazide (co-beneldopa) or carbidopa (co-careldopa). Benserazide and carbidopa do not cross the blood–brain barrier and, therefore, do not interfere with the conversion of levodopa to DA in the basal ganglia. Apomorphine must be administered subcutaneously, and tends to be used in patients with severe 'on-off' fluctuations. Trihexyphenidyl (benzhexol) and benzatropine have anticholinergic effects, and can be used as an adjunct to dopaminergic treatment in patients with prominent tremor. Selegiline selectively inhibits monoamine oxidase B and is used in conjunction with levodopa to reduce end-of-dose deterioration. It may be used as monotherapy, but there is less certainty about its long-term safety profile.

290. A: Graft-versus-host disease

Graft-versus-host disease is caused by donor-derived immune cells-particularly T cells, reacting against the recipient. The incidence increases with age. If it occurs before 100 days it is described as acute and after that as chronic. Acute graft-versus-host disease involves the skin, gut and liver. The skin rash typically involves the palms of the hands and soles of the feet but may involve the whole body. The diagnosis is confirmed by biopsy. The gut manifestations are diarrhoea and vomiting. Typically, the liver enzymes show elevation of the bilirubin and ALP with relatively normal levels of the other enzymes. Chronic graft-versus-host disease typically follows from the acute form and involves the skin, oral mucosa, lacrimal glands, the joints, and other serosal surfaces. The problem is prevented by immune suppression, including ciclosporin, methotrexate, corticosteroids and T-cell depletion. Should it occur, then treatment is with corticosteroids or antilymphocyte globulin (ALG).

291. A: Extrinsic allergic alveolitis (EAA)

EAA and sarcoidosis tend to occur in never- or ex-smokers. LCH, DIP, RB-ILD and CFA are all associated with cigarette smoking. These relationships are not mutually exclusive but make certain diagnoses more or less likely depending on the smoking history.

292. D: Sjögren's syndrome (SS)

Sjögren's syndrome should be considered in a patient with a highly positive rheumatoid factor and no clinical evidence of rheumatoid arthritis. SS is a chronic inflammatory disorder of exocrine glands, leading to dryness and discomfort of the eyes, mouth and vagina. Patients with dry eyes (keratoconjunctivitis sicca) will complain of sensations of grittiness or burning. Patients will frequently describe a scratchy or sandy sensation of the eyes. Contact lenses are poorly tolerated. SS may exist as a primary disorder or can be associated with other autoimmune diseases such as rheumatoid arthritis, systemic lupus erythematosus and systemic sclerosis. Elevation of the erythrocyte sedimentation rate is almost a universal finding in these patients. The presence of rheumatoid factor in up to 80% of these patients suggests that this condition is indeed an immune complex disease. Antibodies to SSA and SSB are more specific serologic markers of SS. There is no clinical or laboratory evidence to suggest SLE or RA as an alternative diagnosis in this patient. Polymyalgia rheumatica is characterised by pain and stiffness around the shoulder and pelvic girdles. Positive rheumatoid factor is not a feature of this disorder. Furthermore it is very rare before the age of 50. Fibromyalgia is a non-inflammatory disorder and, by definition, patients with the disease have normal ESR levels.

293. E: Increased risk of *Salmonella* gastroenteritis

Proton pump inhibitors (PPIs), e.g. omeprazole, reduce gastric acid secretion by 99.0–99.9% and therefore increase gastric pH by 2–3. Adverse effects include rash, impaired liver biochemistry, gynaecomastia and Stevens-Johnson syndrome. The reduction in gastric acid secretion substantially lowers the bacterial threshold required to cause *Salmonella* gastroenteritis. Ferrous sulphate is absorbed best in the ferrous (Fe^{2+}) rather than the ferric form (Fe^{3+}) and its absorption is thus promoted by gastric acid or reducing agents such as ascorbate. Preclinical studies had suggested an increased risk of gastric carcinoma, but this has not been borne out in practice. However, there is concern that gastric carcinoma may present later because symptoms can be masked by the use of PPIs.

294. B: Rheumatoid arthritis

Iritis, visual impairment and even blindness are not uncommon features of many forms of arthritis and rheumatic disease. Joint disorders often associated with iritis include arthritidies related to human leukocyte antigen B27 (HLA-B27), namely the seronegatine spondyloarthropathies, such as ankylosing spondylitis, enteropathic arthropathy, Reiter's syndrome, and psoriatic arthritis. On the other hand, in seropositive disorders such as RA the eye lesions are confined to the conjunctiva/sclera. Iritis is infrequent. Behçet's disease is a rare disorder of oral and genital ulcers, inflammatory eye disease and skin lesions. It causes acute non-granulomatous iritis. Eye involvement is the most serious symptom in Behçet's patients. It occurs in 70% of patients, and 25% will go blind. Between 30% and 40% of patients with sarcoidosis will develop eye problems. The most common is acute or chronic relapsing iritis. Syphilis and tuberculosis could lead to chronic granulomatous iritis and arthritis.

295. E: Randomised placebo-controlled trial in healthy volunteers

In any 'entry in human' (EIH) study trials are conducted in healthy volunteers to assess clinical safety. Each volunteer normally receives only a single dose of drug and studies involve a progressive increase in dosage: this is a 'single ascending dose' study design and is used to detect any major effects of the drug on vital signs or haematological or biochemical or ECG variables. Often, several volunteers in each group will receive placebo. The gold standard study design for optimal quality results is a randomised, double-blind, placebo-controlled study. In phase 1 studies, healthy volunteers are studied, rather than patients. An exception is where the potential risks of the investigational drug are too high to justify administration in healthy people, for example in the development of chemotherapy agents.

296. C: Gingival hyperplasia and zidovudine (AZT)

Antiretroviral treatment involves a combination of two, or ideally three, different drugs, aiming to reduce viral load as much as possible. The major classes of antiviral treatments active against HIV infection are protease inhibitors (PIs), nucleoside reverse transcriptase inhibitors (NRTIs) and non-nucleoside reverse transcriptase inhibitors (NNRTIs). PIs (e.g. saquinavir) are associated with lipodystrophy, hyperlipidaemia, insulin resistance and hyperglycaemia. NNRTIs also have metabolic adverse effects, and nevirapine is associated with a high incidence of Stevens-Johnson syndrome.

297. D: Reduced effectiveness of diuretic treatment

Hepatic impairment is associated with fluid overload, oedema, and ascites. Drug absorption from the gastrointestinal tract may be impaired due to gut oedema, but reduced metabolic capacity can substantially reduce drug metabolism and first-pass metabolism. Generally, there is an overall increase in drug bioavailability. Hypoalbuminaemia leads to a reduction in protein binding, and toxicity can occur due to the increased proportion of free drug. The alterations in fluid status aggravate the effects of diuretic treatment. Patients with hepatic impairment show increased sensitivity to oral anticoagulants because synthesis of clotting factors is already reduced.

298. B: Commence simvastatin

This is an unequivocal indication for statin therapy. After an acute stress event cholesterol measurements may be artificially lowered but not raised: a high reading remains significant. In a patient with end-organ disease any cholesterol over 5.2 mmol/l would be regarded as requiring treatment by all authorities. Many would argue that all post-infarction patients should be commenced on statin therapy regardless of cholesterol measurement.

299. C: Lifestyle advice and recheck blood pressure in six months

This man's second blood pressure reading is only marginally above the 145/85 mmHg threshold for primary prevention. Furthermore, he has at least two lifestyle factors (weight and alcohol excess) that could be modified and would almost certainly reduce his blood pressure. A watching brief and lifestyle advice is merited.

300. C: Patent foramen ovale

The most likely diagnosis is a patent foramen ovale. This can be confirmed with bubble echocardiography (not part of the routine transthoracic echocardiogram). Carotid stenosis is possible, but less likely, and may be non-atheromatous in this age group. Atrial fibrillation rarely leads to embolic phenomena in young people with structurally normal hearts. A subarachnoid haemorrhage may present with sensorimotor deficits, but these are usually less transient and associated with other features such as headache, vomiting and syncope. The story is quite unlike pulmonary embolism.

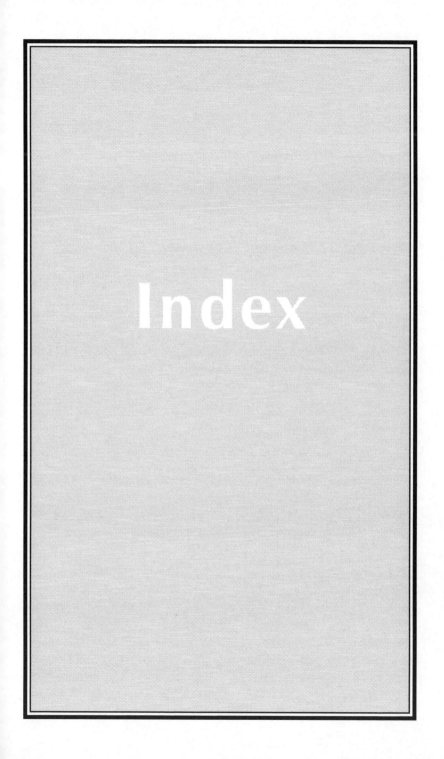

Index

Locators are question/answer number

abciximab 54
abscesses 166, 276, 284
ACE inhibitors 203, 251
aciclovir 197
acne 70
acoustic neuroma 230
acromegaly 214
activated partial thromboplastin time 40
alcohol 29, 74, 245
aldosterone 43, 46
allopurinol 273
alopecia 45, 226
aluminium 207
ambylopia 245
amenorrhoea 107
amiodarone 150
amphotericin 105
anaemia 6, 19, 60, 77, 96, 109, 143, 157, 181, 205, 207, 241, 252
angina 212
ankylosing spondylitis 188
anterior interosseous nerve 187
antibiotics 15, 24, 75, 91, 110, 137, 139, 146, 193, 259
antipsychotic drugs 49, 160
anxiety disorders 23, 196
aorta 249
arthritis 12, 25, 66, 133, 173, 216, 256, 280
ascites 121, 198
aspirin 52, 165
asthma 51, 91, 114, 200, 210, 270, 277
atenolol 138, 225
atherosclerosis 1, 298
atrial fibrillation 14, 156, 163
atrial septal defects 90, 300
autoantibodies 40, 53, 155, 162, 243, 292

back pain 88, 124, 134, 188
bisphosphonates 274
bites 193

blisters 29, 106
blood chemistry 10, 27, 37, 52, 259
blood gases 11, 51, 265
blood pressure *see* hypertension
blood transfusions 32, 47
brain
    benign intracranial hypertension 99
    infarctions 44, 72, 113, 218, 271
    infections 7, 164, 166, 218, 219
    parietal lesions 44, 72, 122
    space occupying lesions 3, 20
breastfeeding 151
Brown-Séquard syndrome 282
bulimia nervosa 171
bumetanide 191

calcium 94, 235, 247
calcium-channel blockers 177, 190, 225
carbon monoxide poisoning 265
cardiopulmonary exercise test 100
catecholamines 154
cerebellar ataxia 21
chickenpox 264
cholesterol 204, 298
chronic obstructive pulmonary disease (COPD) 123, 186, 222
Churg-Strauss syndrome 76, 243
ciprofloxacin 75
cirrhosis 69, 198, 221, 288
clinical trials 295
Clostridium difficile 15, 110
clozapine 49, 160
coagulation disorders 40, 54, 129, 278
cognitive impairment 122
colitis 15, 110, 236
colorectal cancer 56
constipation 152
contraception 70, 285
copper 170
coronary arteries 202
corticosteroids 43, 127, 158, 209, 210, 222, 274
cortisol 43, 127, 236, 240, 270

heart disease
  arrhythmias 14, 42, 67, 79, 126,
      156, 163, 176, 211
  drugs 28, 150, 163, 177, 189, 190,
      191, 203, 212, 225, 238, 250,
      257
  infective 26, 50, 139, 224, 248
  ischaemic 1, 116, 135, 212, 238,
      298
  myxoma 283
  restrictive 269
  septal defects 90, 300
Helicobacter pylori 184
hemiparesis 14, 156, 300
Henoch-Schönlein purpura 5
hepatitis 35, 193, 268, 272, 288
herpes simplex virus 7, 61
hirsutism 2
HIV 115, 128, 161, 175, 192, 287,
    296
HLA genes 188
Hodgkin's disease 263
hormone replacement therapy 261
hydrocortisone 43, 127, 236, 240, 270
hydroxychloroquine 216
hyperimmune immunoglobulin 234
hypertension 46, 99, 103, 121, 154,
    198, 203, 225, 299
hyperviscosity syndrome 120
hypoglycaemia, non-diabetic 71
hypoglycaemic agents 83, 141, 194
hypomania 217
hyponatraemia 10, 27
hypotension 246, 249

immune reconstitution illness 128
immunosuppressants 281
inotropic agents 163, 177, 189, 190,
    203, 225, 250
iron 60, 173, 195
ischaemia, TIAs 14, 156, 300
isotretinoin 70

jaundice 35, 47, 142, 259
jaw claudication 223

keratoderma 117, 167

kidney
  biopsy 140
  calculi 65, 235
  cysts 78, 164
  diabetic complications 118, 251, 258
  dialysis 197, 207, 247, 267
  mesangial IgA disease 168, 183
  nephritis 108, 130, 149, 162, 220,
      272
  nephropathy 149, 275, 287
  pharmacokinetics 104
  renal failure 162, 206, 220, 258
  renal tubular acidosis 37
  transplants 92
Koebner phenomenon 153

leishmaniasis 105
leptospirosis 206
leukaemia 85
leukaemoid reaction 215
lithium 68
liver
  abscesses 276, 284
  drugs 95, 259, 297
  metabolic disorders 13, 170
  primary sclerosing cholangitis 41
  transplants 142
  see also cirrhosis; hepatitis
lung disease
  cancer 161
  COPD 123, 186, 222
  cryptogenic fibrosing alveolitis 11
  diagnosis 76, 100, 131, 201, 232,
      267, 291
  embolism 237, 279
  hypertension 103
  infections 24, 50, 115, 119, 146,
      201, 209
  interstitial 254
  sarcoidosis 39
  SLE 101
  see also asthma
Lyme disease 82
lymphadenopathy 228, 263

medicolegal issues 135
megacolon 152

PASTEST BOOKS FOR MRCP PART 1

At PasTest we are continually updating our books to reflect changes in the Part 1 examination. We provide up-to-the-minute material in all specialties to give the busy MRCP 1 candidate essential practice before sitting the examination.

Essential Revision Notes for MRCP: Revised Edition
P Kalra FRCP RCP Tutor   1 901198 59 6
A definitive guide to revision for the MRCP examination. 19 chapters of informative material necessary to gain a successful exam result.

MRCP 1 'Best of Five' Multiple Choice Revision Book
K Binymin MBChB MRCP MSc   1 901198 57 X
Over 300 'Best of Five' questions and expanded answers. Subject-based chapters reflecting the actual exam content to test your knowledge and highlight weak areas for further revision.

Essential Lists for MRCP
S McPherson BSc MBChB MRCP et al   1 901198 58 8
This book is a compilation of clinical, diagnostic, investigative and prognostic features of the symptoms and diseases that cover the whole spectrum of general medicine.

MRCP 1 Pocket Book Series
Each pocket-sized book contains 50% of 'Best of Five' questions on popular Membership topics with detailed teaching notes
Book 1: Cardiology, Haematology, Respiratory Medicine   1 901198 75 8
Book 2: Basic Sciences, Neurology, Psychiatry   1 901198 80 4
Book 3: Endocrinology, Gastroenterology, Nephrology   1 901198 85 5
Book 4: Clinical Pharmacology, Immunology, Infectious Diseases,
        Rheumatology   1 901198 90 1

MRCP 1 BASIC MEDICAL SCIENCES: Second Edition
P J Easterbrook MRCP & J Greenwood MBChB MRCP   1 901198 93 6
A second edition of this popular title has been adapted to Best of Five format questions. The book contains 300 exam-based questions and detailed answers arranged by subject.

MRCP Part 1 MCQ Key Topic Summaries: Second Edition
P O'Neill MRCP   1 901198 07 3
This book bridges the gap between standard question and answer books and textbooks. Each question has a comprehensive key topic summary to aid revision.

Essential Statistics for Medical Examinations
B Faragher PhD FSS & C Marguerie MRCP   0 906896 82 7
Essential information for candidates taking medical examinations at all levels.
This book covers all aspects of statistical methodology commonly tested in medical examinations.

HOW TO ORDER:

www.pastest.co.uk
To order books safely and securely online, shop online at our website.

Telephone: +44 (0) 1565 752000
Make sure you have your credit card to hand when you call.

PasTest Ltd, FREEPOST, Knutsford, WA16 7BR
Send your order with a cheque (made payable to PasTest Ltd). Please put your address details on the reverse of the cheque.

Fax to +44 (0) 1565 650264
Fax your order with your debit or credit card details.

Delivery to your Door
With a busy lifestyle, nobody enjoys walking to the shops for something that may or may not be in stock. Let us take the hassle and deliver direct to your door. We will dispatch your book within 24 hours of receiving your order.